Critical Care Ultrasound for Emergency Situations and Clinical Applications

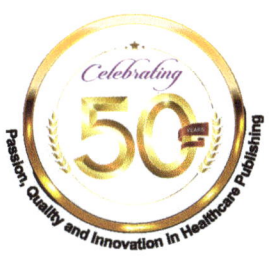

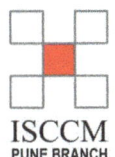

ISCCM
PUNE BRANCH

Critical Care Ultrasound for Emergency Situations and Clinical Applications

Editors
Pradeep D'Costa
DNB (General Medicine) Certificate in Critical Care (ISCCM)
Head
Department of Critical Care Medicine
KEM Hospital and Research Center
Senior Faculty
Sahyadri Hospital (Shastri Nagar Branch)
Pune, Maharashtra, India

Jayant Shelgaonkar
MBBS DA MD FRCA (UK) FICCM
Head
Department of Critical Care
Jupiter Hospital
Pune, Maharashtra, India

Foreword
Shirish Prayag

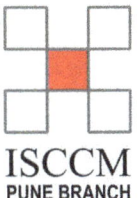

ISCCM
PUNE BRANCH

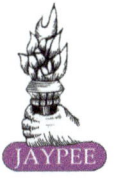

JAYPEE

JAYPEE BROTHERS MEDICAL PUBLISHERS
The Health Sciences Publisher
New Delhi | London | Panama

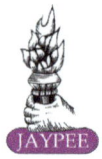 **Jaypee Brothers Medical Publishers (P) Ltd.**

Headquarters
Jaypee Brothers Medical Publishers (P) Ltd.
4838/24, Ansari Road, Daryaganj
New Delhi 110 002, India
Phone: +91-11-43574357
Fax: +91-11-43574314
Email: jaypee@jaypeebrothers.com

Overseas Offices

JP Medical Ltd.
83, Victoria Street, London
SW1H 0HW (UK)
Phone: +44 20 3170 8910
Fax: +44 (0)20 3008 6180
E-mail: info@jpmedpub.com

Jaypee-Highlights Medical Publishers Inc.
City of Knowledge, Bld. 235, 2nd Floor, Clayton
Panama City, Panama
Phone: +1 507-301-0496
Fax: +1 507-301-0499
E-mail: cservice@jphmedical.com

Jaypee Brothers Medical Publishers (P) Ltd.
Bhotahity, Kathmandu, Nepal
Phone: +977-9741283608
E-mail: kathmandu@jaypeebrothers.com

Website: www.jaypeebrothers.com
Website: www.jaypeedigital.com

© 2020, Jaypee Brothers Medical Publishers

The views and opinions expressed in this book are solely those of the original contributor(s)/author(s) and do not necessarily represent those of editor(s) of the book.

All rights reserved. No part of this publication may be reproduced, stored or transmitted in any form or by any means, electronic, mechanical, photocopying, recording or otherwise, without the prior permission in writing of the publishers.

All brand names and product names used in this book are trade names, service marks, trademarks or registered trademarks of their respective owners. The publisher is not associated with any product or vendor mentioned in this book.

Medical knowledge and practice change constantly. This book is designed to provide accurate, authoritative information about the subject matter in question. However, readers are advised to check the most current information available on procedures included and check information from the manufacturer of each product to be administered, to verify the recommended dose, formula, method and duration of administration, adverse effects and contraindications. It is the responsibility of the practitioner to take all appropriate safety precautions. Neither the publisher nor the author(s)/editor(s) assume any liability for any injury and/or damage to persons or property arising from or related to use of material in this book.

This book is sold on the understanding that the publisher is not engaged in providing professional medical services. If such advice or services are required, the services of a competent medical professional should be sought.

Every effort has been made where necessary to contact holders of copyright to obtain permission to reproduce copyright material. If any have been inadvertently overlooked, the publisher will be pleased to make the necessary arrangements at the first opportunity. The **CD/DVD-ROM** (if any) provided in the sealed envelope with this book is complimentary and free of cost. **Not meant for sale.**

Inquiries for bulk sales may be solicited at: jaypee@jaypeebrothers.com

Critical Care Ultrasound for Emergency Situations and Clinical Applications

First Edition: **2020**

ISBN: 978-93-86261-03-8

Dedicated to

My daughter Anandini and wife Shalini, and full family. Without whose support it would have been impossible to complete.

Pradeep D'Costa

Contributors

J Chacko MD DNB EDIC MBA
Consultant and Head
Critical Care Services
Narayana Multispeciality Hospital
Bengaluru, Karnataka, India

Pradeep D'Costa
DNB (General Medicine)
Certificate in Critical Care (ISCCM)
Head
Department of Critical Care Medicine
KEM Hospital and Research Center
Senior Faculty
Sahyadri Hospital (Shastri Nagar Branch)
Pune, Maharashtra, India

Deepak Govil
Director
Critical Care Medicine
Medanta—The Medicity
Gurugram, Haryana, India

Srishti Jain
EDIC–European Diploma in Intensive Care Medicine
FNB–Critical Care (Mumbai)
MD–Pulmonary Medicine (Gold Medalist)
DNB–Respiratory Diseases
EDARM–European Diploma Respiratory Medicine
DAA–Diploma Allergy and Asthma
Assistant Professor
Department of Critical Care
Mahatma Gandhi Medical College and Hospital
Jaipur, Rajasthan, India

Sachin Jagdale
FCPS (General Medicine)
Diploma Critical Care (ISCCM)
Senior Intensivist
KEM Hospital and Research Center
Pune, Maharashtra, India

Arindham Kar
MD DNB FNB EDICM FCCP, FICCM, FCCM
Director and HOD
CK Birla Hospitals
CMRI Institute of Critical Care
Kolkata, West Bengal, India

Valentine Lobo
MD (Medicine) DNB (Nephrology)
Consultant Nephrologist
King Edward Memorial Hospital
Mumbai, Maharashtra, India

Rahul Pandit
MD FJFICM FCICM EDICM FCCP FICCM DA
Director
Department of Critical Care
Fortis Hospital, Mulund
Mumbai, Maharashtra, India

Pratibha Patel
MBBS DA IDCCM
Critical Care Consultant
KEM Hospital
Pune, Maharashtra, India

Manish Pathak
MBBS DA FCPS IDCCM
In-charge
Transplant Anesthesia and Critical Care
Sahyadri Group of Hospitals
Pune, Maharashtra, India

Vrushali Ponde MD DA
Consultant Pediatric Anesthesiologist
Director
Children Anesthesia Services
Surya Children Hospital
Mumbai, Maharashtra, India

Jayant Shelgaonkar
MBBS DA MD FRCA (UK) FICCM
Head
Department of Critical Care
Jupiter Hospital
Pune, Maharashtra, India

Shrikanth Srinivasan
Consultant and Head
Critical Care Medicine
Manipal Hospital
New Delhi, India

Ashish Srivastava
Consultant
Critical Care Medicine
Manipal Hospital
New Delhi, India

Kedar Toraskar
Consultant Intensivist and Pulmonologist
Wockhardt Hospital
Mumbai, Maharashtra, India

Charudutt Vaity
MD DNB MRCP (UK) EDIC MFICM (UK)
Senior Consultant
Department of Critical Care
Fortis Hospital, Mulund
Mumbai, Maharashtra, India

Ravindra Zore
MD (General Medicine)
Consultant Intensivist
Wockhardt Hospital
Mumbai, Maharashtra, India

Foreword

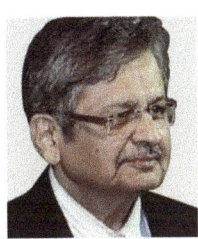

It is with a great degree of pleasure and pride that I am writing this Foreword. 25 years ago, there was no organized professional activity although isolated foci of excellence in critical care existed in India in individual centers. Training in this evolving field was nonexistent. It is then in 1992, that an organized platform for discussions in small group was started in Pune, Maharashtra, under the banner of Critical Care Society. In 1993, the Indian Society of Critical Care Medicine (ISCCM) was born and this local activity in Pune merged with ISCCM as its first city branch.

Over the past 25 years of activity, Pune Branch of ISCCM has remained in the forefront of academic activities of ISCCM and the critical care world in India. There have been innumerable activities, and all this has led to Pune being awarded the Best Branch award for many consecutive years.

We have always believed in giving something different, unique and enriching to the world of critical care in India. The workbooks for various workshops are therefore a part of this continuing process of dynamic output from this branch.

The field of ultrasonographic imaging has advanced very rapidly over the last three decades. It is a very unique imaging tool due to its portability, widespread availability and safety. Hence, it comes as no surprise that the advances in this field have overlapped the branch of Critical Care Medicine. As it stands today, it is an indispensable modality of evaluating the critically-ill patient. So much so that its utility is perhaps more than the stethoscope.

The range of its utility has been quite staggering and hence a number of well-designed courses have evolved for the benefit of the trainees in critical care medicine. Today, you cannot expect to do a critical care training without training in sonology.

This workbook is a reflection of the needs of the new trainees and the advances and expertise available. I am sure that it will be an important companion to the resource material for trainees in critical care medicine.

Shirish Prayag MD FCCM
Director
Department of Critical Care
Prayag Hospital
Pune, Maharashtra, India

Preface

It is indeed a proud moment for us!

We will be releasing one of the first books on Critical Care Ultrasound in India.

The "Specialty" of Critical Care Ultrasound has now taken firm roots in India.

We will be entering nearly a decade of Critical Care Ultrasound in our country soon.

Gone are the days when we viewed ultrasound as a fearful and completely mysterious area. The apprehensions of the past have been replaced by hope, joy and fulfilment after utilizing the ultrasound almost by the hour to make critical lifesaving decisions in our units and hence improve the quality of care as well as the accuracy and safety of our clinical decision making.

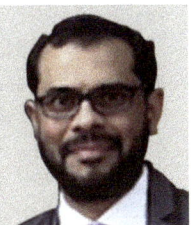

Pradeep D'Costa

With many recommendations coming in fields like vascular access guidance, lung ultrasound, procedural guidance, in trauma by focused assessment with sonography in trauma (FAST)/ extended focused assessment with sonography in trauma (EFAST), in cardiac arrest situations suggesting ultrasound use in our ICUs, it may also be medicolegally incorrect not to give our patients the benefits of this technology in the future!

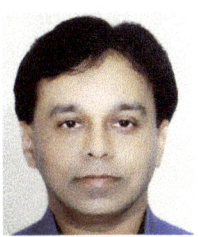

Jayant Shelgaonkar

The "Pune" group of World Interactive Network Focused On Critical UltraSound (WINFOCUS) have the proud privilege of being the first ITU (International training unit) to be recognized in the country for training in Critical Care Ultrasound. This honor was bestowed on us at the Rome world conference of WINFOCUS in 2010.

Our mentor Dr Luca Neri deserves our sincere acknowledgments and praise for the massive role he has played, in addition to other heavyweights like Dr Daniel Lichteinstein, Dr Enrico Storti, Dr Gabriele Via, without whose help and guidance expanding the horizons in our country would have been difficult.

The beginnings for us as a team were since around 2008, those were the days where the "phobia" for using ultrasound was still high, and machines to use and practice and train were indeed sparse.

Indeed since then, the interest and applications of this fascinating specialty have grown, new applications are being found very regularly, new uses with profound clinical implications are there to be discovered and worked upon…

This workbook has made a sincere effort to first put forth the basics in particular areas of critical care along with the clinical implication in critical or emergency care.

The authors themselves are well-known experts in their respective fields and their experience too can be noted and felt here.

The present book intends to cover the basics and will take you on a quick "round" of the ICU, from the basic physics (relevant to emergency settings), airways and the applications, a section dedicated to the lungs and new uses including acute respiratory distress syndrome (ARDS) management, the heart and clinical applications for the intensivist.

Trauma, vascular access, and nerve blocks in addition to a special section on transplant related ultrasound (since the number of transplants will only increase in coming years posing many critical care-related issues), as also a section on critical care nephrology applications.

We have added a special section on various procedures that can be done in the emergency settings as well.

An upcoming section, that of neurocritical care uses of the ultrasound makes its way into the book.

We would like to reinforce however, that this technology is by no means a substitute to clinical examinations of patients or special lab tests. Indeed the maximum benefits would be delivered to the patients if we utilize the total knowledge (clinical + ultrasound + lab) as a robust comprehensive care package!

This book is just an appetizer of the things to come, as in the coming years we plan to add sections on orthopedic applications, applications of the skin and subcutaneous tissues as well as sections on obstetric emergencies.

We hope you enjoy reading the book and give us valuable suggestions for improvement.

Using this knowledge (of ultrasound in emergency settings) to possibly save a life will indeed be a purpose well served in writing the book!

Pradeep D'Costa
Jayant Shelgaonkar

Acknowledgments

We, on behalf of the Pune branch of the Indian Society of Critical Care Medicine (ISCCM), appreciate and value the contribution of all the authors who have made contributions.

We acknowledge their chapters and indeed their valuable inputs provided on sometimes difficult to write topics, and hope the readers' benefits much from their rich experience.

We are grateful to Shri Jitendar P Vij (Group Chairman), Mr Ankit Vij (Managing Director), Ms Chetna Malhotra Vohra (Associate Director–Content Strategy) and Ms Nedup Denka Bhutia (Development Editor) of M/s Jaypee Brothers Medical Publishers (P) Ltd, New Delhi, India, has been very patient with us and deserve a special commendation. The work they are doing in spreading this knowledge is indeed great and heartening.

We are obliged to Dr Kapil Zirpe who has been backing us fully in this project, and has given us a free hand, truly to be appreciated.

We are thankful to our local coordinator, Archana who has been helpful in coordinating amongst various persons.

Lastly, we must acknowledge our mentor and friend Dr Luca Neri, whose teachings, vision, guidance and experience has helped us make this humble attempt of the book!

Contents

1. **Introduction to Critical Care Ultrasound and Clinical Implications** — 1
   Pradeep D'Costa

2. **Basic Ultrasound Physics for the Critical Care Fellow** — 4
   Jayant Shelgaonkar

3. **Ultrasound of the Airways for Emergencies** — 20
   Shrikanth Srinivasan, Deepak Govil, Ashish Srivastava

4. **Ultrasound of the Lung and Clinical Uses in Emergencies** — 31
   Pradeep D'Costa

5. **Focused Cardiac Ultrasound** — 49
   J Chacko, Jayant Shelgaonkar, Rahul Pandit, Charudutt Vaity

   Part 1: Focused Cardiac Ultrasound for the Acute Care Physician—Basic Views, Anatomy, and Measurements
   J Chacko

   Part 2: Focused Hemodynamic Assessment at Bedside—Interpretations, Fluid Management, and Basic Eyeballing Principles
   Jayant Shelgaonkar

   Part 3: Critical Care Ultrasound—Valvular Assessment, Regional Wall Assessment, and Diastolic Dysfunction Assessment
   Charudutt Vaity, Rahul Pandit

6. **Abdominal Aortic Aneurysm, Deep Vein Thrombosis and Pulmonary Embolism: Use of Ultrasound** — 83
   Srishti Jain, Ravindra Zore

7. **Ultrasound of the Gallbladder, Pancreas and Bowel in Emergencies** — 93
   Pratibha Patel

8. **Ultrasound Use in Nephrology, Critical Care Settings and Post-transplant Period** — 105
   Valentine Lobo, Arindham Kar

9. **Role of Ultrasound in the Liver Transplant Patient** — 115
   Manish Pathak

10. **Ultrasound in the Neurocritical Care Setting** — 117
    Pradeep D'Costa, Kedar Toraskar

11. **Ultrasound in Trauma (FAST/eFAST in Trauma Victim)** 140
    Pratibha Patel

12. **Ultrasound-guided Vascular Access** 160
    Sachin Jagdale

13. **Ultrasound-guided Nerve Blocks: Basics** 175
    Vrushali Ponde

14. **Ultrasound-guided Procedures** 188
    Kedar Toraskar

Index *199*

CHAPTER 1

Introduction to Critical Care Ultrasound and Clinical Implications

Pradeep D'Costa

INTRODUCTION OF CRITICAL CARE ULTRASOUND

The word ultrasound has been in use for some time now.

In the late 1700's echolocation in bats was studied. After nearly a century thence, Curie brothers discovered the phenomenon of piezoelectricity, the princilple of which is still utilised for the ultrasound probes.

Interestingly, the *Titanic* tragedy too has a bearing on ultrasound, as it was after this tragedy that Langevin invented a hydrophone (possibly the first known transducer) to find articles at the bottom of the sea!! The early 1900's saw use in the field of sports (to ease pains in footballers! detecting brain tumors, detect gall stones, detect breast tumors). Since the discovery of ultrasound and its potential uses, as had been studied in bats, we have indeed come a long way.

The initial units were quite bulky and indeed very discomforting for the subject, the uses being only in a select few, which since then have changed.

Previously considered the realm of only highly-specialized radiology experts, now has made way to experts from a wide variety and backgrounds making full use of this new technology (emergency, surgeons, orthopedicians, gynecologists, neurologists and intervention specialists).

POCUS or point of care ultrasound is the new term coined for ultrasound done at the direct point of care i.e., at the bedside of the patient. This "bedside" would include critical units, emergency departments, operation theaters, outpatient units as well as situations on the field like trauma victims, roadside accident victims, war situations and also severely austere situations like mountains, snow, sports field, etc. The widespread outreach has been so extensive that we now even have POCUS been done in space stations!!!!

As you may guess the outreach is tremendous and the potential is great!

Just consider a situation of a medical emergency in a very remote area of our country, let us say a trauma situation in shock, and we require to take a decision about operating room or shifting to a higher center.

A quick-fast examination by ultrasound, either interpreted on the spot or by telemedicine by experts sometimes sitting miles away or indeed continents away, can help in making crucial decisions and hence save the life!!

The beginning of POCUS was indeed, as many would say, during the Vietnam war. It was used to good effect to save war victims.

During the early 80's pioneering work was done in this field by Prof. Daniel Lichtenstein.

He explored the lungs considered the graveyard for the sonologist and indeed also by prominent authors like Harrison (medicine), he covered the whole body and changed the scene forever. It is not without reason, he is known widely by many as the father of modern day POCUS. Later prominent bodies like WINFOCUS (World Interactive Network Focused On Critical Ultrasound) have helped to disseminate this knowledge to many countries and indeed to the resource poor areas as well (Brazil project).

The earlier uses of POCUS were in vascular access and conventional abdominal ultrasound as also with diagnosing gynecological emergencies. We have come a long way since then.

We now can approach the patient in a complete head to toes manner in an emergency situation.

A wide-range of structures can be evaluated by the use of ultrasound. Brain-brain substance, midline shifts, fractures, pupils, transcranial Doppler for monitoring patients of subarachnoid hemorrhage (SAH), and also helping to diagnose severely-injured brains and aid in brain death diagnosis. Sinuses, orbits, cervical spine area, neck, airways, esophagus, lungs, abdomen, including liver, kidneys, bowels, spleen, pancreas all are well visualized. The heart is seen in a totally different perspective by the point-of-care cardiac ultrasound, many decisions like fluid management, lines, pacing can be done. A good visualization of aorta, veins of the central circulation, and peripheral ones, too make the use more interesting.

In addition to this, a whole variety of procedures are now done bedside under direct ultrasound guidance, making all these procedures much more safe and accurate. Procedures like vascular access (both veins and arteries), nerve blocks, fluid tapping, drain insertions, transvenous pacing, drug injections and lumbar punctures can indeed be done with improved safety.

Unfortunately, in countries like India, strict acts governing ultrasound use are in place, which sometimes limit or restrict the use.

Acts like PCPNDT (Pre-Conception and Pre-Natal Diagnostic Techniques Act, 1994) which have been put in place to prevent female feticide has important benefits preventing the abuse of the ultrasound machine and indeed protecting the unborn child, but this also prevents liberal and free use of the machine and technology by wider sections of the emergency personnel, including paramedical or nonmedical staff.

We must have a good knowledge of these acts, its provisions and also its translations in clinical practice to be able to benefit our patients with most accuracy. Local authorities and hospital administrators must be taken into confidence, every time a new machine is procured or new users are added to the existing machine, and appropriate protocols prescribed by the authorities have to be followed stringently to avoid any medicolegal problems (including sealing of machines and legal action including jail). The authorities also require regular updating of the clinical activities by filling certain forms which must be done with due diligence and care as many a time even clerical errors are looked upon very strictly.

There are however many new applications which are being discovered regularly (transcranial Doppler, new procedures, lung classifications) which make this new field a very promising and fascinating one! Portability of these machines (much less bulky and smaller) now makes them easily transportable, to even remote locations and situations, and thus prove as invaluable tools to save lives.

Truly the modern day stethoscope is indeed the ultrasound probe!!!

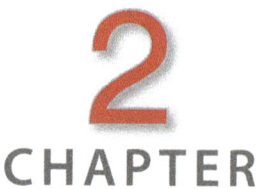

Basic Ultrasound Physics for the Critical Care Fellow

Jayant Shelgaonkar

INTRODUCTION

Sound wave is a mechanical wave that travels in a straight line in a medium. It is heard by human ear when it travels through the air at an audible frequency. Frequency of audible ultrasound ranges between 20 Hz and 20,000 Hz. Waves produced by ultrasound usually are above are 20,000 Hz. These are inaudible to the human ear. Ultrasound used for diagnostic purposes ranges between 1 MHz and 10 MHz.

Ultrasound has several characteristics that contribute to its diagnostic utility.
- It can be focused accurately on specific areas of interest and be directed as a beam
- Physical properties like reflection and refraction are followed by ultrasound waves as it traverses a medium
- Even small objects tend to reflect the waves and can be picked up and described. However, ultrasound waves do not travel through a gaseous medium.

An ultrasound wave travelling through a medium produces vibration of particles in the medium parallel to the line of the wave (longitudinal waves). These longitudinal movement of wave in the medium produces alternate areas of compression and rarefaction. How the sound wave behaves (by reflection, refraction or attenuation) depends on the acoustic properties of the medium through which it passes. Targets containing solid material, very dense areas tend to reflect significant ultrasound energy, and cause poor tissue penetration. Ultrasound waves pass through soft tissues, blood and fluid without or minimum attenuation hence the echoes reflected from the structures distal to it are stronger which improves visualization of the structure being examined. Bones also reflect more ultrasound waves because it has increased density and multiple interfaces.

To understand various terminologies we draw a sound wave on the graph which looks like a "sine wave". It contains peaks and low areas called troughs which signify the compression and rarefaction respectively. One compression wave and one rarefaction wave constitutes one wave cycle. A wavelength is defined as the distance between two consecutive points along the wave. If the wavelength increases, frequency reduces and if frequency increases wavelength reduces.

Wavelength affects axial resolution of the image, hence lesser wavelength, hence higher frequencies, causes better resolution but less penetration. So, probes with higher frequency (5–10 MHz) give better resolution and hence are used to study superficial structures like vessels, nerves and are as also useful in children.

Probe

Probes with low frequency (2–5 MHz) have better penetration but at the cost of resolution, hence are used for deeper structures like abdominal organs. Sound waves travel through different mediums at different velocities, called the propagation velocity. This velocity again depends on the denseness and compressibility of the medium. Tissue hardness is directly proportional to this propagation velocity (Fig. 2.1 and Table 2.1). The average velocity of the sound wave in the body 1,540 m/s.

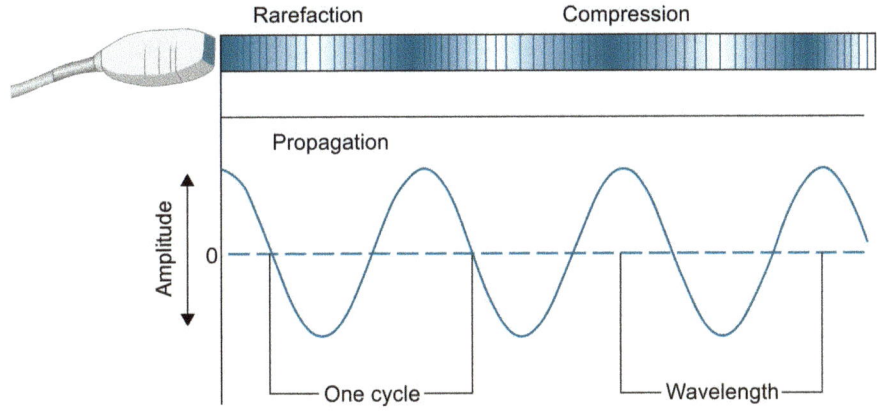

Fig. 2.1: Propagation velocities.

Table 2.1: Various propagation velocities.	
Substance	Velocity in (m/s)
Air	330
Fat	1,450
Water	1,480
Soft tissue	1,540
Renal	1,560
Blood	1,570
Muscles	1,580
Bones	4,080

TRANSDUCERS

The essential element of each ultrasound transducer is a piezoelectric crystal, serving both to generate, and to receive ultrasound waves.

The ultrasound transducers differ in construction according to:
- Piezoelectric crystal arrangement
- Footprint
- Operating frequency (which is directly related to the penetration depth).

The following types of transducers are most often used in the critical ultrasound imaging:

Sector (Fig. 2.2):
- Piezoelectric crystal arrangement—phased array (most commonly used)
- Footprint size—small
- Operating frequency (bandwidth)—1-5 MHz (usually 3.5-5 MHz)
- Ultrasound beam shape—sector, almost triangular
- Use—small acoustic windows, mainly echocardiography, gynecological ultrasound, and upper body ultrasound.

Linear (Fig. 2.3):
- Piezoelectric crystal arrangement—linear
- Footprint size—usually big (small for the hockey transducers)
- Operating frequency (bandwidth)—3-12 MHz (usually 5-7.5 MHz)
- Ultrasound beam shape—rectangular
- Use—ultrasound of the superficial structures, e.g. obstetrics ultrasound, breast or thyroid ultrasound, vascular ultrasound.

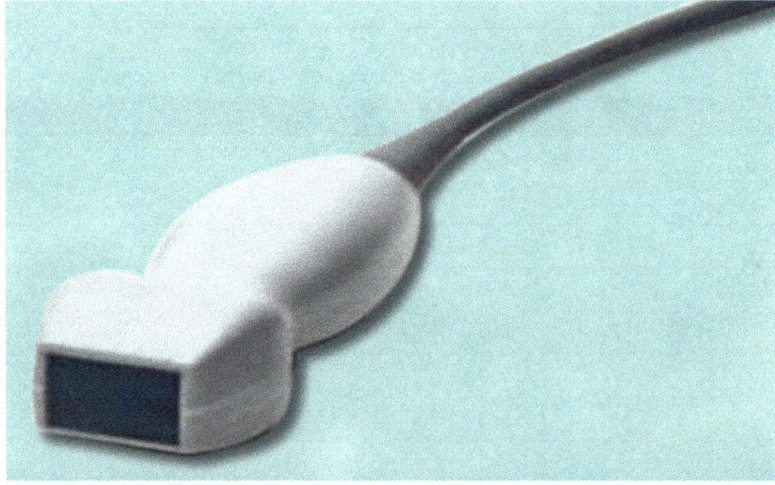

Fig. 2.2: Transducers.

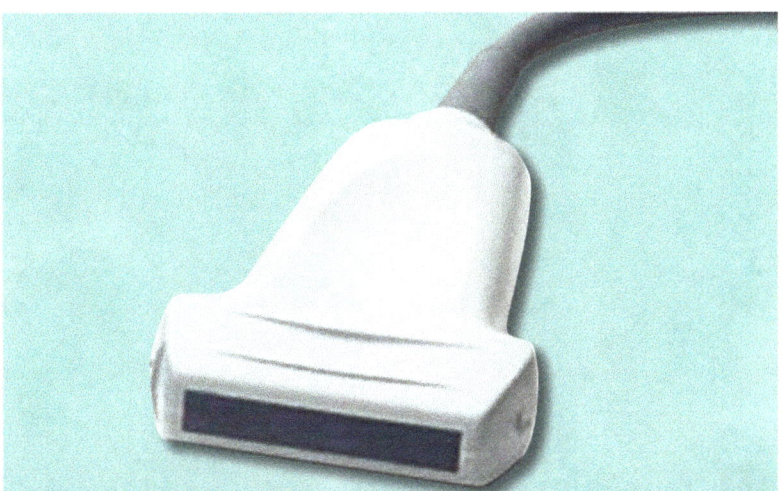

Fig. 2.3: Linear.

Convex or microconvex (Figs. 2.4A and B):
- Piezoelectric crystal arrangement—curvilinear, along the curvature
- Footprint size—big (small for the microconvex transducers)
- Operating frequency (bandwidth)—1–5 MHz (usually 3.5–5 MHz)
- Ultrasound beam shape—sector; the ultrasound beam shape and size vary with distance from the transducer that causes the lack of lateral resolution at greater depths
- Use—useful in all ultrasound types except echocardiography, typically abdominal, pelvic, and lung (microconvex transducer) ultrasound.

Attention!

An ultrasound transducer is the most important and usually the most expensive element of the ultrasound machine, so it should be used carefully, which means the following:
- Do not throw, drop, or knock the transducer
- Do not allow to spoil the transducer's duct
- Wipe the gel from the transducer after each use
- Do not sluice with alcohol-based preparations.

Beam

The ultrasound transducer has multiple piezoelectric crystals, which emits the ultrasound waves. The beam is formed by these waves and happens as close to the horizontal plane as possible.

Orientation

Each transducer usually has a prominent dot or an illuminating source or a mark, which assists the user in the orientation process. There is also a mark on the ultrasound machine screen to help the user to get oriented with the images.

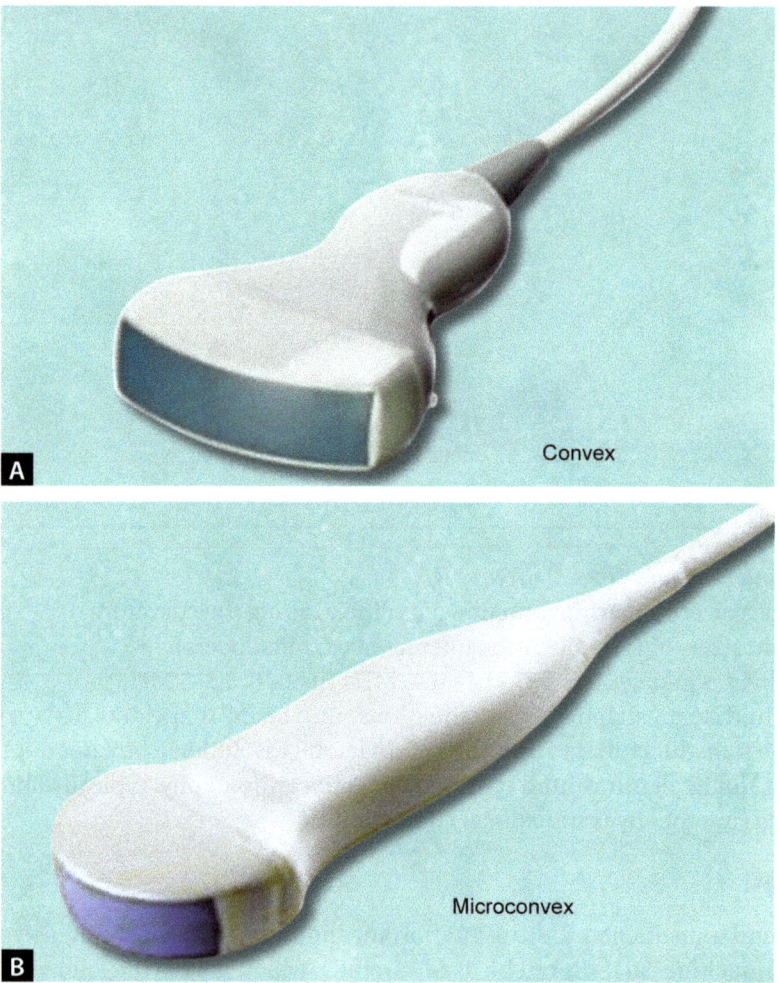

Figs. 2.4A and B: Convex or microconvex.

Interaction between Ultrasound and Tissue

When an ultrasound wave passes through the tissue, its energy is attenuated or weakened. This loss of intensity or energy of an ultrasound wave is due to its properties of reflection, absorption, scattering phenomenon, and refraction phenomena.

Reflection

"Acoustic impedance" is the measure of opposition that a tissue presents to the acoustic flow i.e. propagation speed. It also depends on the properties of two adjacent tissues. If the two adjacent tissues have same acoustic impedance values, no echoes will be produced at its interface. But if the acoustic impedance values of two adjacent tissues having dissimilar properties are different, an echo will be produced at its interface. If the difference is minute, a low intensity or weak echo is produced, and if acoustic impedance variation is big, a stronger echo will be generated. If the difference in acoustic impedance is very large, all the ultrasound waves will be totally reflected. Typically in soft tissues, the amplitude of an echo produced at a boundary is only a small percentage of the incident amplitudes, whereas areas containing bone or air reflect almost all of the incident ultrasound waves producing large echoes that not enough ultrasound remains to image beyond the tissue interface. At a tissue–air interface, 99% of the beam is reflected, so none is available for further imaging. To reduce this reflection of beam at skin air interface, we use gel between the probe and the skin. The ultrasound waves also obey the law of reflection. The angle of incidence produced by US waves with the tissue is equal to angle of reflection. We need to keep in mind when we are performing ultrasound examination. It we hole the transducer at an angle less than 90, the echoes will be reflected away from the transducer. Hence to obtain a clear image we should always work or hold the transducer perpendicular to the structure being examined (Fig. 2.5).

Scattering

Some of the echoes are reflected back to the probe and some are scattered in all directions in a non uniform manner. This is especially true for very small objects or rough surfaces. The part of the scattering that goes back to reach the transducer and generate images is called back scatter.

Absorption

During transmission of an ultrasound wave in the tissue, its energy gets absorbed and this contributes most to the attenuation of an ultrasound wave in tissues.

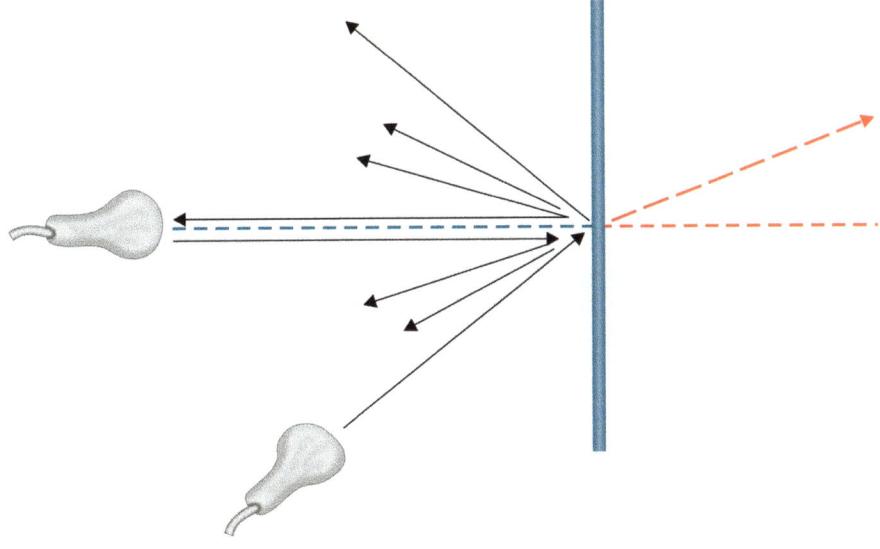

Fig. 2.5: Reflection.

Refraction

When the ultrasound wave traverses the tissue, there is change in the direction of a sound wave at tissue interface at an oblique angle to the tissue interface. This is called as refraction.

RESOLUTION

It is the ability of the ultrasound machine to distinguish between two objects, which are in close proximity.

Axial resolution: It is the ability of the ultrasound machine to identify two objects, which are lying close to each other as two objects along the axis of the ultrasound beam. Axial resolution depends on the wavelength of an ultrasound. Higher frequency transducer will emit ultrasound waves with small wavelengths giving better the axial resolution (Fig. 2.6).

Lateral resolution: It is the ability of an ultrasound machine to distinguish two objects as two objects which are perpendicular to the direction of the beam. It depends on the width and thickness of the beam, distance from the transducer. Lateral resolution decreases as width of the beam increases (Fig. 2.7).

Temporal resolution: It is the ability of an ultrasound machine to detect moving objects in the field of view in their true sequence. The number of frames generated per second (frame rate) determines temporal resolution.

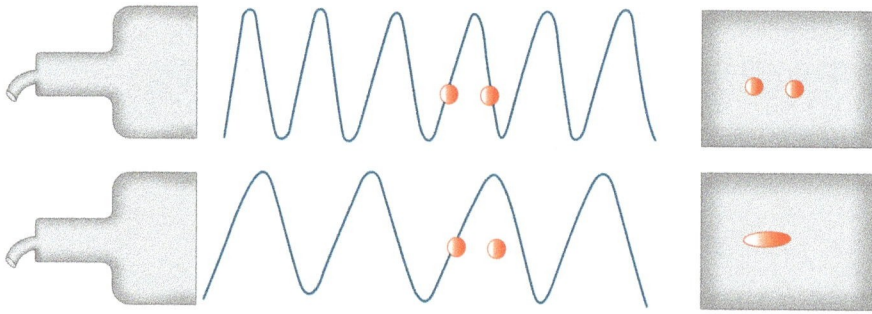

Fig. 2.6: Axial resolution.

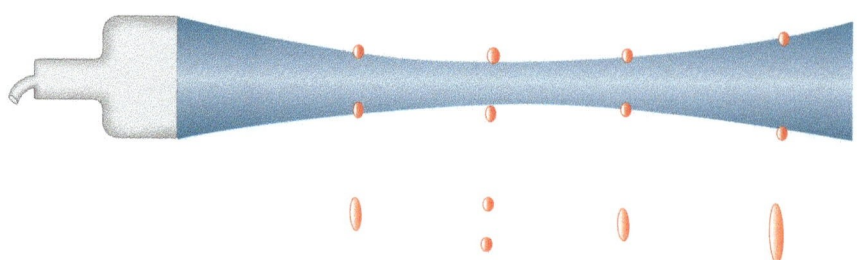

Fig. 2.7: Lateral resolution.

Contrast resolution: It is ability to distinguish and display different shades of grey within the image.

MODES OF ULTRASOUND

Various modes are used to study different structures.

A Mode

It is also called "amplitude modulation" mode. It displays reflected echoes as amplitudes of different heights depending on its strength. This mode is used in ophthalmology to measure the axial length (Fig. 2.8).

B Mode

Also called brightness mode or brightness modulation. It is the most common form of mode used on the ultrasound machines. It displays two-dimensional cross-sectional view of the structures being examined. The returning echoes are displayed as bright spots on the screen and the intensity of these bright spots depend on the strength of returning echo. There are no amplitudes seen in this mode and does not have a Y-axis representation, but a Z-axis (echo intensity) and X-axis (depth). Hence, we do not get vertical spikes in this mode (Fig. 2.9).

M Mode

This is also called time motion or TM or motion mode. Used commonly for cardiac purposes, it analyses moving body parts in a one dimensional mode or image over a time period. Initially

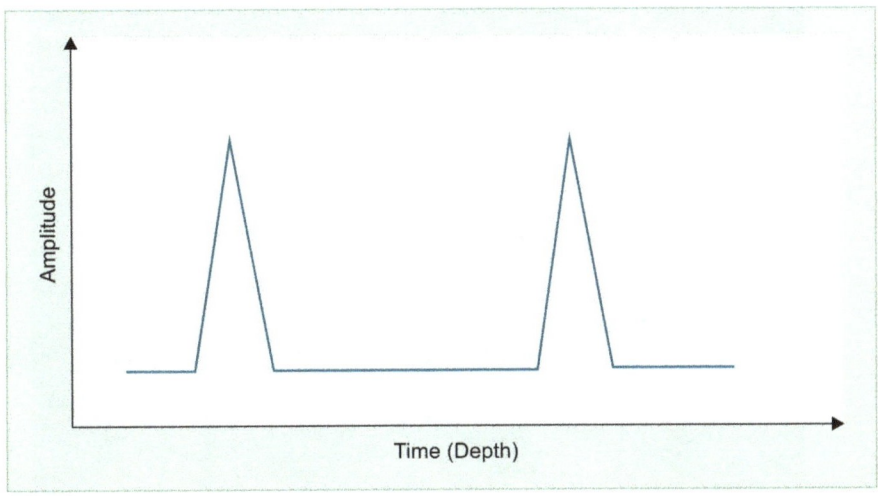

Fig. 2.8: A Mode.

2D image is acquired and a single scan line or a beam is placed across the area of interest. Echoes reflected by the structures intersected by this beam are displayed as dots of varying intensities creating a lines across the screen (Fig. 2.10).

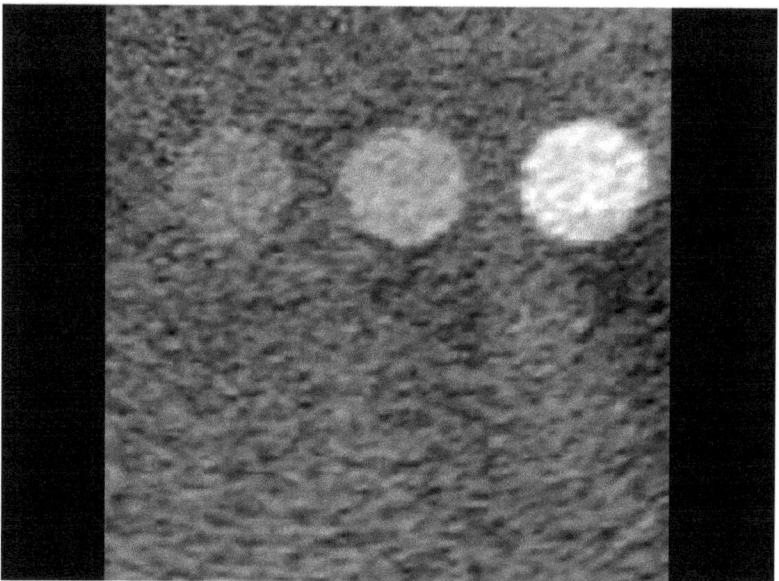

Fig. 2.9: B Mode.

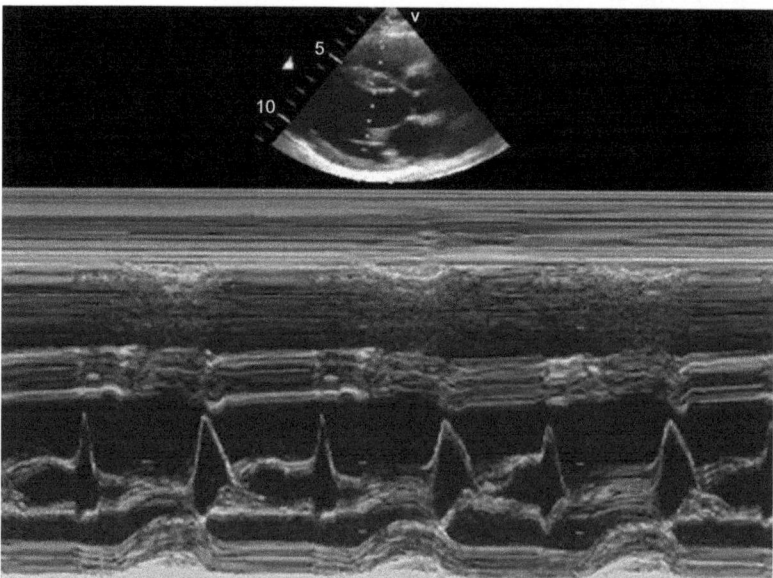

Fig. 2.10: M Mode PLAX view.

TISSUE HARMONIC IMAGING

When the ultrasound wave is transmitted in the body, the fundamental frequency of the echo signal may be altered because of its nonlinear interaction with the tissue. This interaction results in the generation of frequencies which are not present in original ultrasound wave. These new frequencies are called harmonics. The strength of the harmonic frequency increases as the wave penetrates deep inside the body as opposed to the fate of fundamental frequency wave which attenuates during propagation. Tissue harmonic imaging reduces artifact generation as weak fundamental signals produce almost no harmonics because most of the artifact result from weak fundamental signals.

DOPPLER ULTRASOUND

Doppler imaging is concerned with the movement of a target in relation to the transducer. This phenomenon was studied by Austrian physicist Christian Doppler in 1842. He observed that as the source of sound moved towards the listener, the frequency and pitch of the sound increased. Conversely if the source of sound moved away from the listener, the frequency and the pitch of the sound decreased. This increase or decrease in frequency due to relative motion between the transducer and the target is known as "Doppler shift".

He also described the relationship between the magnitude of the frequency shift and the velocity of the target and the angle between the interrogating beam and the flow ($\Delta f \alpha v x \cos \theta$).

The value of cosine of 0° is 1. That means a measured velocity is the true velocity when there is no angle between the blood flow and the beam. As the angle between the blood flow direction and the beam increases from 0° to 90° the cosine θ decreases from 1 to 0. For any angle more than 0 there is decrease in calculated velocity. For practical purposes this decrease in calculation of velocity becomes significant when the angle increases more than 20°.

There are five Doppler techniques:
1. Continuous wave Doppler
2. Pulsed wave Doppler
3. Color flow imaging
4. Tissue Doppler
5. Duplex scanning.

Pulse Wave Doppler

Pulse wave (PW) Doppler measures velocity at single point. The US is transmitted in the body in intermittent bursts. It transmits and then goes into listening mode to receive reflected signals. Although targets at multiple points along the beam reflect the transmitted ultrasound, the PW Doppler listens to a signal at a specific depth chosen by the operator. It samples the velocity of blood at that point. PW Doppler has a major drawback that it cannot correctly depict higher velocities (usually above 1.5–1.7 m/s). Aliasing is commonly seen with pulse wave Doppler.

Continuous Wave Doppler

In continuous wave Doppler the signal is transmitted and received continuously. In phased array transducer one crystal is dedicated for transmitting while other is simultaneously receiving the signal. One of the major advantage of continuous wave Doppler is imaging is that aliasing does not occur and very high velocities can be accurately measured. It samples everything along the line.

Color Flow Imaging

It is a two-dimensional display of intracardiac velocities. It is also a pulse wave Doppler technique, hence gives us a depth acuity and is unable to measure high velocities. Each pixel in the two-dimensional image acts as a small pulsed Doppler sample volume and displays the movement of blood as a colored dot. Blood moving toward the transducer is represented as shades of red, and blood moving away from the transducer is depicted as shades of blue. Turbulent (nonlaminar) blood flow is represented by the addition of green hues to the other colors (a mosaic pattern). Aliased velocities shift the color from red to blue or vice versa (color reversal).

Tissue Doppler Mode

Tissue Doppler is an application of Doppler principle. By adjusting gain and reject setting, this technique is used to document the motion of the muscles of the heart rather than blood. Blood has a much higher velocity than tissue; hence, we adjust the machine to get the lower velocity ranges. Tissues are strong reflectors of Doppler signal hence some additional adjustments are required to avoid oversaturation. This tissue Doppler imaging is used to derive the velocity information.

ARTIFACTS

Artifacts are errors in image formation. These are normally caused by physical processes that affect the ultrasound. We must keep in mind that there are certain basic assumptions made during the analysis of reflected echoes and production of an ultrasound images.
- The sound wave can travel in a straight line, and reflects from all structures, which are present in the central axis of the wave.
- Sound waves travel (1,540 m/s) to and from this reflecting surface.
- The ability of the reflecting medium to reflect waves (reflector scattering strength) governs the intensity of this reflection.
- The attenuation of sound in tissue does not vary.
- All detected echoes originate from the axis of main beam only.
- All received echoes are derived from the most recently transmitted pulse.

These artifacts are generated during an imaging may actually provide useful information about the area being examined and help us in interpreting the anatomy or an abnormality in that area.

Main artifacts seen in critical care of clinical significance are:
- *Reverberation artifact*
  - In this artifact, the wave bounces back and forth (reverberate) between the 2 reflectors which are parallel to each other. US assumes that an echo returns to the transducer after a single reflection and that the depth of an object is related to the time for this round trip. In the presence of two parallel highly reflective surfaces, the echoes generated from a primary ultrasound beam may be repeatedly reflected back and forth before returning to the transducer for detection. When this occurs, multiple echoes are recorded and displayed. The echo that returns to the transducer after a single reflection will be displayed in the proper location. The sequential echoes will take longer to return to the transducer, and the ultrasound processor will erroneously place the delayed echoes at an increased distance from the transducer. At imaging, this is seen as multiple equidistantly spaced linear reflections and is referred to as reverberation artifact. Changing the angle of interrogation will help minimize or remove the artefact and can improve the image quality (Fig. 2.11).
  - These artifacts can be divided into:
    - *Comet-tail artifact:*
      - In this artifact, the two reflective interfaces are closely spaced and hence the sequential echoes are also closely spaced. On the screen, the sequential echoes may be so close together that individual signals are not perceivable. In addition, the later echoes may have decreased amplitude secondary to attenuation and gradually they become less echoic (Fig. 2.12).

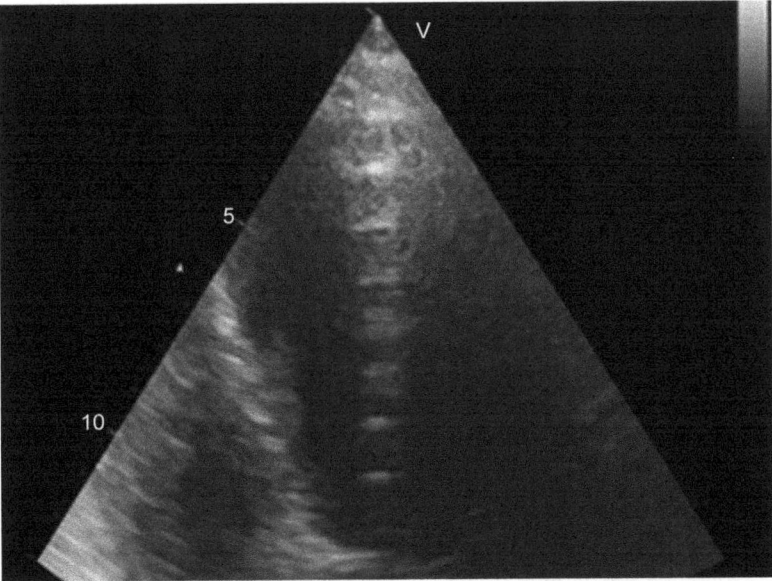

Fig. 2.11: Reverberation artifact.

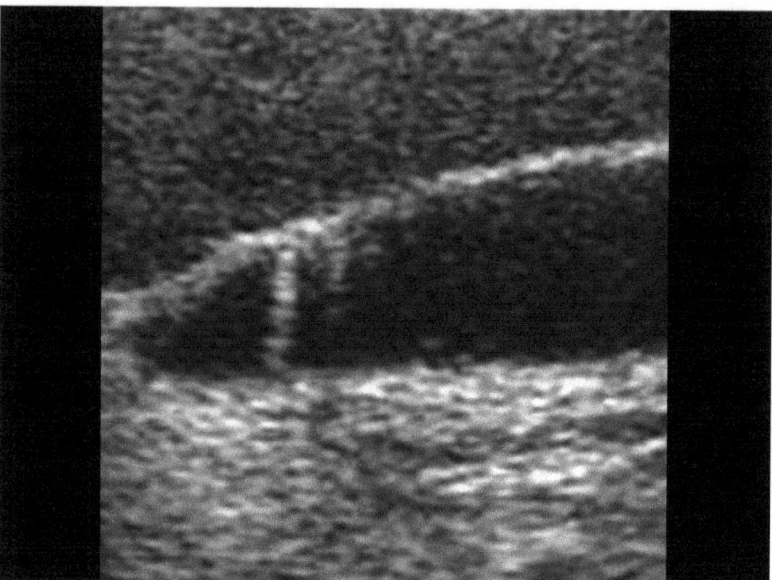

Fig. 2.12: Comet tail artifact.

- *Ring down artifact:*
    - In the past this ring down artefact was thought of as a variant of comet tail artefact as both appeared similar. But now we know it has a separate mechanism. The transmitted ultrasound energy causes resonant vibrations within fluid trapped between a tetrahedron of air bubbles. These vibrations create a continuous sound wave that is transmitted back to the transducer. This phenomenon is displayed as a line or series of parallel hyperechoic bands extending posterior to a gas collection (Fig. 2.13).
- *Acoustic shadowing*
    - This phenomenon is seen with a strong reflector. When the wave reflects of this surface, the amplitude of the beam distal to this strong reflector is diminished. The echoes returning from structures beyond the highly attenuating structure will be diminished. As a result of this the structures lying distally may be missed or not seen. This is seen on the screen as a dark or hypoechoic band known as a "shadow" deep to a highly attenuating or reflective structure (Fig. 2.14).
- Enhancement artifact
    - When the ultrasound beam encounters a weakly attenuating structure within the imaging field, the amplitude of the beam beyond this structure is greater than the beam amplitude at the same depth in the rest of the field. Hence the echoes returning from structures deep to this weak attenuator will be of higher amplitude giving us enhanced view. On the display, we see hyperechoic signals extending from an object of low attenuation. This artifact can be used by the clinician to narrow a differential diagnosis (Fig. 2.15).

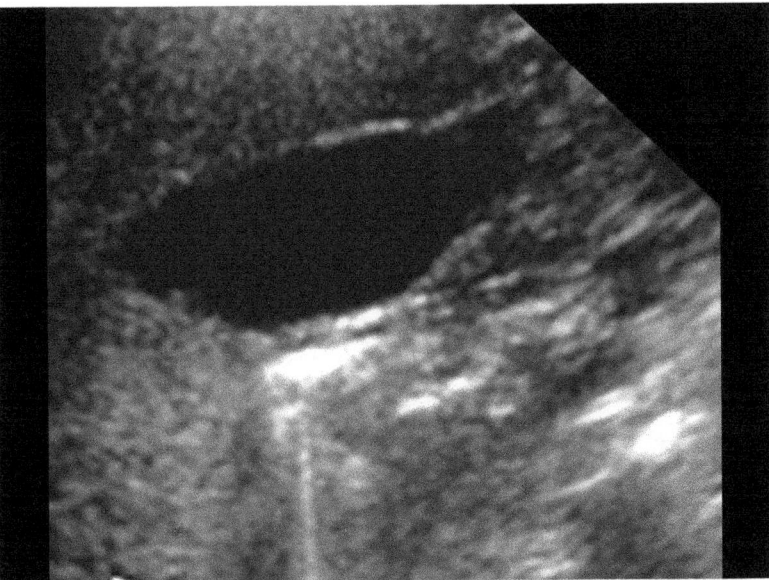

Fig. 2.13: Ring down artifact.

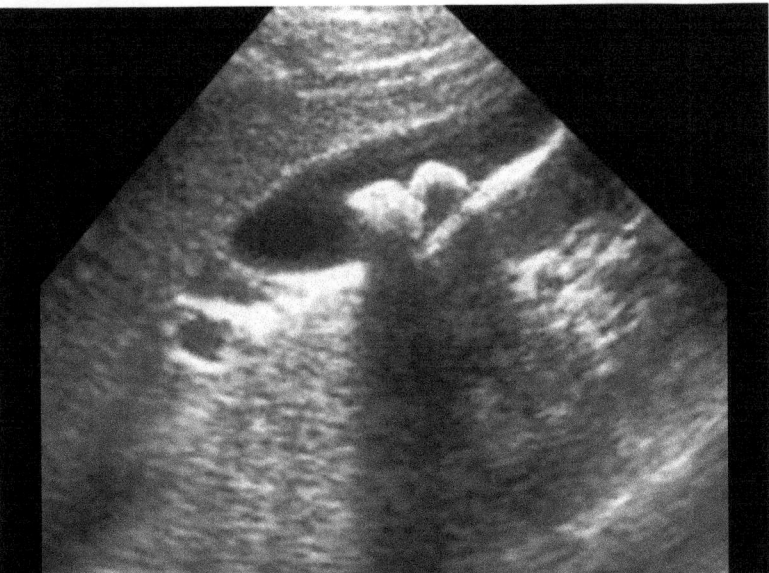

Fig. 2.14: Acoustic shadowing.

- Mirror image artifact
    - Mirror image artifacts is generated when a primary beam encounters a highly reflective surface like diaphragm. Some echoes are reflected towards the transducer but some encounter the structure and are reflected back toward the reflective interface before being

reflected to the transducer for detection. The machine assumes that an echo returns to the transducer after single reflection and the ultrasound beam travels in a straight line. As a result the display shows a duplicated structure or the mirror image of that structure equidistant from but deep to the strongly reflective interface (Figs. 2.16 A and B).

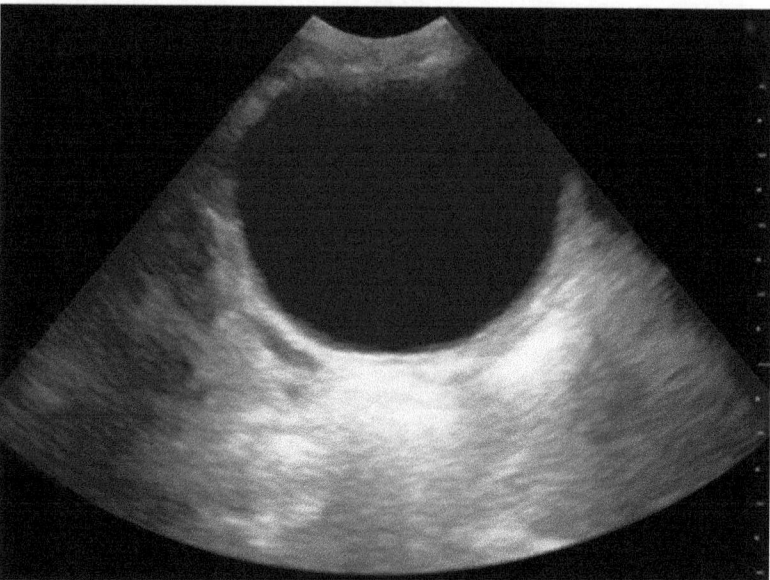

Fig. 2.15: Enhancement artifact.

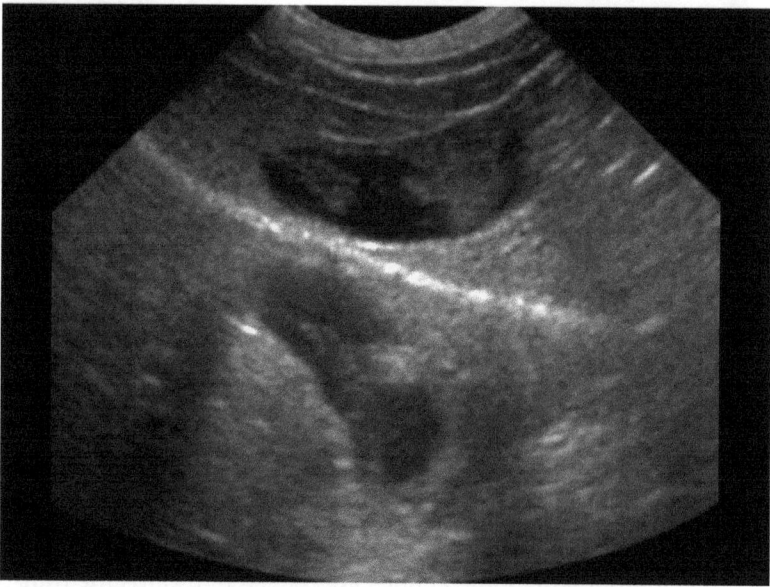

Figs. 2.16A

Basic Ultrasound Physics for the Critical Care Fellow

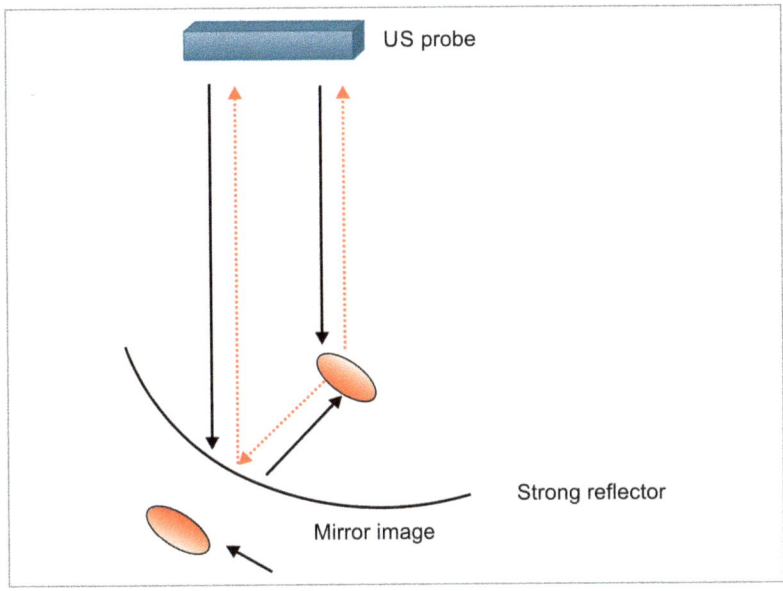

Figs. 2.16B

Figs. 2.16A and B: Mirror image artifact.

SUMMARY

In conclusion, point-of-care ultrasound is an important tool to examine, diagnose, and the medical condition. Its utility at the bedside is just now being recognized. Understanding the physics of sound waves and how the system generates images is important in acquiring the best possible images to aid in diagnosis and management.

SUGGESTED READING

1. Edelman SK. Understanding ultrasound physics. Texas: ESP; 2005.
2. Shriki J. Ultrasound Physics. Crit Care Clin. 2014;30:1-24.
3. William FA, Ryan T, Feigenbaum H. Feigenbaum's Echocardiography, 7th Edition. Philadelphia: Lippincott Williams & Wilkin; 2010.
4. Zagzebski JA. Essentials of ultrasound physics. United States: Mosby; 1996.

Ultrasound of the Airways for Emergencies

Shrikanth Srinivasan, Deepak Govil, Ashish Srivastava

INTRODUCTION

Point of care ultrasound (POCUS) is an invaluable noninvasive, bed side tool for the physician to detect pathology, monitor and follow-up disease conditions real time, and with a high level of accuracy.

Point of care ultrasound-guided upper airway assessment is a useful adjunct for airway management even when the anatomy is distorted due to trauma or disease conditions, the use of ultrasound gives us valuable information regarding upper airway structures like epiglottis, thyroid cartilage, vocal cords, cricoid cartilage (CC), cricothyroid membrane (CTM), tracheal rings, and also the esophagus.

Knowledge of this enables the clinician to use the ultrasound machine in cases of difficult intubation, accurate endotracheal tube (ETT) placement, as also laryngeal mask airway (LMA) placement.

In children it helps us also to get the proper size of ETTs.

The applications are also utilized to guide emergency procedures like cricothyroidotomy, tracheostomy, as well as in the postextubation period to predict stridor, as well as to detect upper airway pathologies.

In this chapter we shall discuss the utility of POCUS of upper airway in emergency settings.

APPLIED SONOANATOMY OF THE UPPER AIRWAY

For proper interpretation of images produced, we require to have a very basic knowledge of image generation, proper selection of the probe as also a basic knowledge of applied anatomy, relevant to the critical care setting.

Position of the Patient

The subject usually is placed in the supine position, placing a padding or pillow under the occiput region (for appropriate head extension and neck flexion). Some describe this as the "sniffing" position.

Transducer

Since structures located in the neck are relatively superficial, we choose the high-frequency linear transducer.

Orientation of the Transducer in the Neck

There are three main ways to orient the probe to visualize the upper airway anatomy (Figs. 3.1A to C):
1. Transverse view (horizontally across the anterior part of the neck)
2. Longitudinal (along the parallel length of the upper airway).
   This can be further divided into:
   - Sagittal view (which is midline and longitudinal)
3. Parasagittal view (which is longitudinally, but lateral to midline).

ULTRASOUND APPEARANCE OF DIFFERENT STRUCTURES IN THE NECK

Air is a poor medium for transmission of ultrasound waves and hence ultrasound cannot visualize the interior of air-filled structures. Whenever, there is air interposed in the path of the ultrasound beam, there is production of artifacts and underlying deeper structures cannot be visualized hence, this air–mucosal (A–M) interface gives a bright (hyperechoic) linear appearance with underlying artifacts. Intraluminal air can give rise to both comet-tail artifacts (CTA), which are vertical, laser like hyperechoic lines and reverberation artifacts which are horizontal repetitive hyperechoic lines.

In the transverse view, the thyroid cartilage is seen as an inverted V-shaped greyish (hypoechoic) structure. The A–M interface can be seen as a bright hyperechoic artifact just beneath the apex of the inverted V-shaped cartilage (Fig. 3.2).

Vocal cord visualization is best done by a transverse view at the thyroid cartilage level. Vocal ligaments produce a hyperechoic appearance, which are seen in the longitudinal views. False vocal cords are located parallel, but slightly cephalad after locating the true cords. On asking the patient to speak, the true cords show dynamic oscillations and move to the midline while the false cords remain relatively still or immobile (Fig. 3.3).

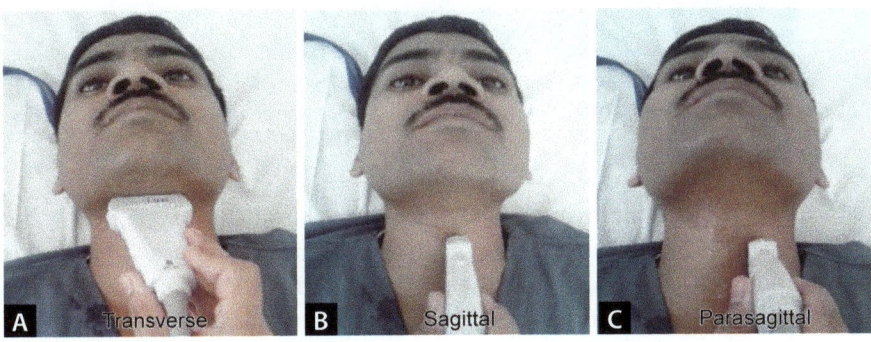

Figs. 3.1A to C: Probe orientation for airway assessment.

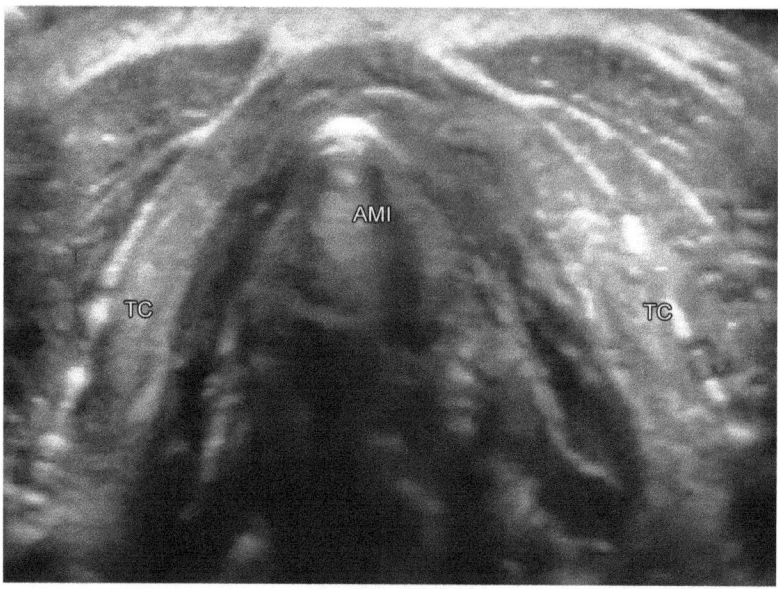

Fig. 3.2: Inverted V-shaped thyroid cartilage (TC) with bright A–M interface (AMI) beneath. (AMI: Air-mucosal interface).

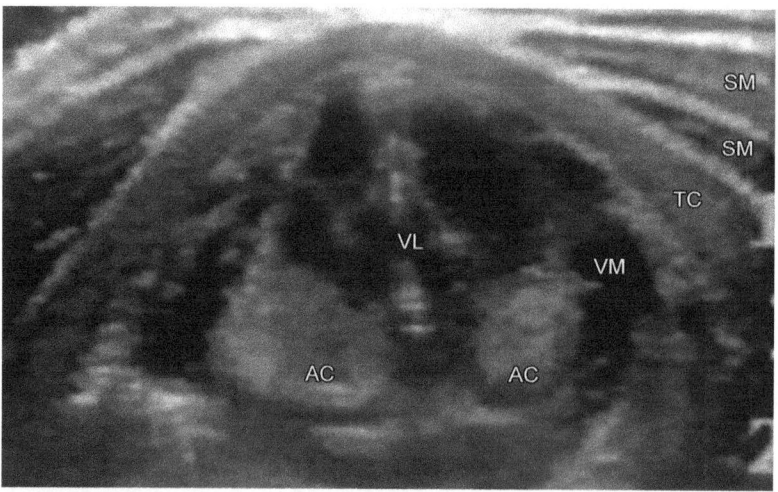

Fig. 3.3: Transverse section through thyroid cartilage (TC) showing hyperechoic vocal ligament (VL), hypoechoic vocalis muscle (VM), arytenoid cartilage (AC), and strap muscle (SM).

The CC can be seen as an inverted U-shape cartilage in the transverse view. It is identified as an oval hypoechoic hump like appearance in the sagittal and parasagittal views. Presence of a bright A–M interface helps us identify the posterior part of the anterior wall of this cricoid as well as intraluminal air, which produces reverberation artifacts (Figs. 3.4A and B).

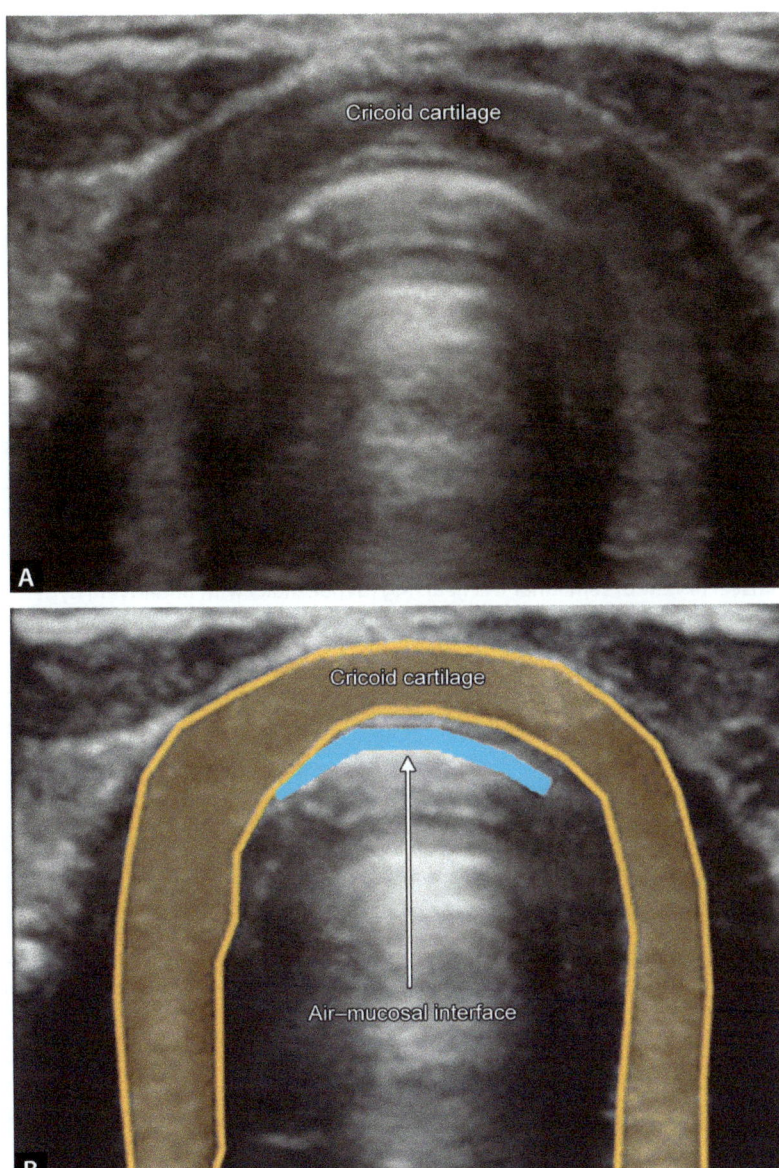

Figs. 3.4A and B: Transverse view of cricoid cartilage with A–M interface (AMI) (AMI: air–mucosal interface).

The tracheal cartilages appear semilunar hypoechoic crescents with a bright A–M interphase below in transverse plane (Fig. 3.5) and in longitudinal plane is seen as a hypoechoic "string of beads" the thick hyperechoic line seen posteriorly on longitudinal view of the trachea is produced by the reverberation artifacts generated by this A–M interface[1,2] (Fig. 3.6).

In the horizontal view, both the lobes of the thyroid gland (TG) can be seen in a position anterolateral to the trachea. Thyroid parenchyma produces a typically homogeneous

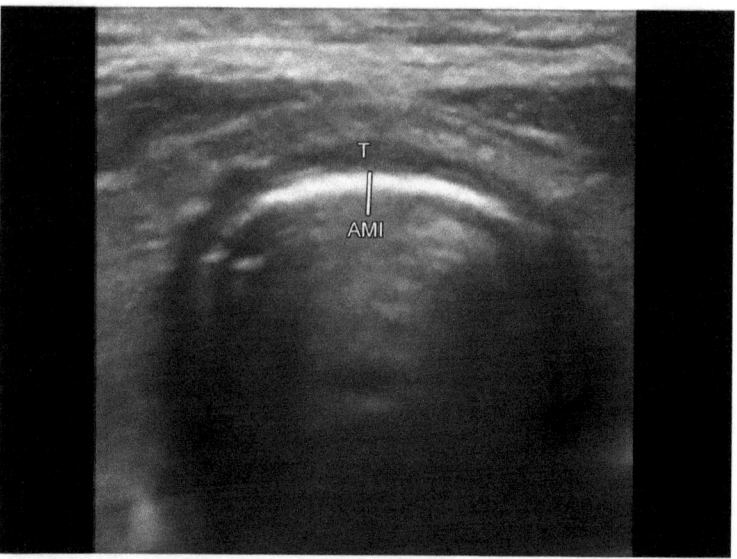

Fig. 3.5: Transverse view of semilunar tracheal ring (hypoechoic) with underlying hyperechoic A–M interface. (AMI: air–mucosal interface).

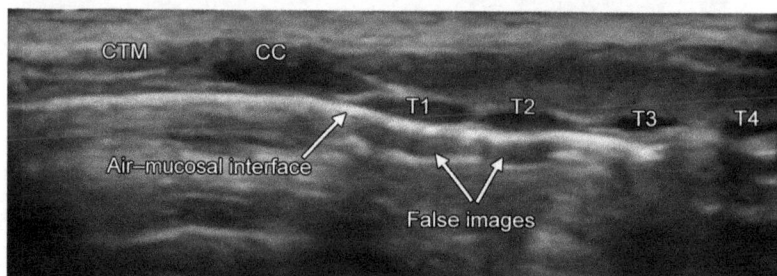

Fig. 3.6: Longitudinal view along trachea showing string of pearls appearance of cricoid cartilage (large round hypoechoic oval) and tracheal rings (smaller ovals) with bright air-mucosal interface beneath with underlying reverberation artifacts.
(CC: cricoid cartilage; CTM: cricothyroid membrane)

ultrasound appearance, which hyperechoic when compared with the adjacent strap muscles.

The esophagus is located in the transverse plane (level at the tracheal cartilages), located posteromedial to the left thyroid lobe. Any Visible dilation and peristaltic movement can be observed within the esophageal lumen during the swallowing act.

Measurement of Subglottic Area Diameter for Choosing and Predicting Endotracheal Tube Sizes

The narrowest diameter of the airways is usually at the postcricoid lumen area (transverse diameter), which can be assessed quite reliably by the use of POCUS. Correlation of reasonably good nature has been documented by comparing the subglottic transverse diameter and the outer diameter of the ETT.[3-5] This has also been confirmed by comparisons with magnetic resonance imaging (MRI) and computed tomography (CT) scans.[6,7]

Lakhal et al.[6] concluded about the similar accuracy of the ultrasound to the MRI in healthy adults when assessing the diameter of the subglottic airway at the cricoid lumen level.

Changes in the laryngeal cartilages in the form of calcifications sometimes begin to appear in the third decade of life, may sometimes limit accurate measurements of subglottic diameters, by creating acoustic shadows.

In the pediatric age group, however, ultrasound measured subglottic airway diameters measured are a reasonably accurate predictor of proper cuffed and uncuffed ETT sizes. Shibasaki et al.[3] measured the subglottic diameter at the lower edge of the CC in patients with controlled ventilation, paralyzed patients and without positive end-expiratory pressure (PEEP).

They concluded that age and height-based formulas can predict accurately only 35% of cuffed ETT size and 60% of uncuffed tube size as compared to a much higher percent when ultrasound is used (98 and 96%, respectively). Hence, in this pediatric subset of patients, this POCUS has been found to be superior to standard age-based and height-based calculations in estimating ETT size.

Identifying of Difficult Situations Prelaryngoscopy in Obese Patients

By measuring volume of anterior neck soft tissues in such subgroup of patients, it is possible to predict a situation of difficult laryngoscopy.

Difficulty in visualization of the hyoid bone by sublingual ultrasound predicts a difficult airway situation with high rate of sensitivity and specificity (Hui et al., positive likelihood ratio of 21.6, negative likelihood ratio of 0.28).[8]

Ezri et al.[9] studied the amount of soft tissues in the pretracheal space, mainly above vocal cords, isthmus of thyroid and suprasternal notch, by measuring the distance from skin to these structures. Amount of soft tissue was calculated by the average in central axis, and 15 mm right, left of central axis.

Patients having more soft tissue (pretracheal, at level of vocal cords found to be more accurate) of 28 mm and larger neck circumference of 50 mm (vocal cord levels) had a difficult time during laryngoscopy.

Adhikari et al.[10] measured the soft tissue thickness anteriorly at hyoid bone level and thyrohyoid membrane level and found good correlations with difficult intubations. Studying independently only the anterior neck soft tissue thickness at thyrohyoid membrane levels may also be used as a separate predictor of a difficult laryngoscopy.

Most of these studies although show promise, but are limited by small sample size and being pilot studies, larger studies have to be undertaken before this modality can become adopted as routine clinical practice.

ENDOTRACHEAL INTUBATION AND DOUBLE-LUMEN BRONCHIAL TUBE PLACEMENT

Ultrasound evaluation with probe placed transversely across the trachea can visualize real time the passage of the endotracheal tube in the trachea. This appears as a transient disturbance of the intratracheal A–M interface as the tube slides into the trachea. Besides this, the lung sliding sign ("to-and-fro" movement of the pleura synchronized with ventilation) can be seen and this is taken as indirect evidence of the correct ETT tube placement in paralyzed or nonbreathing patients. Bilateral active descent of the diaphragm (M-mode) toward the abdomen also gives an idea of accurate placement of the ETT.[11]

In unilateral lung, endobronchial intubation can be identified by watching movement of the diaphragm and occurrence of lung-sliding sign on the ventilated lung (endobronchial) as opposed to absent or very reduced movement of the diaphragm and no lung-sliding sign on the opposite side (no ventilation in lung).[12]

Esophageal Intubation

Accidental esophageal intubation will result in dilation of the otherwise normally collapsed esophagus along with a double ring appearance of tube within it (also called the double tracheal sign) and absence of lung sliding. Ventilation through a malpositioned tube in the esophagus could sometimes result in appearances of paradoxical motion of the diaphragm studied by M-mode, the movements may occur because of raised intra-abdominal pressure or distended stomach caused by excess positive pressure ventilation.[12]

Currently, POCUS is considered a valuable tool to detect endotracheal intubation and accidental esophageal intubation with high degree of accuracy and a small learning curve.[13-15]

Chenkin et al. after a brief online tutorial training (10 minutes) and very few practice attempts (only two) using ultrasound, emergency personnel were able to accurately identify clips of esophageal and endotracheal intubation [one practice attempt (>90%)] and two practice attempts (100%) (Fig. 3.7).[14]

Ultrasound-guided Upper Airway Anesthesia to Facilitate Awake Intubation

By ultrasound, we can identify the superior laryngeal nerve (between the hyoid bone and thyroid cartilage), which can be easily visualized by transverse scan across the hyoid bone. The thyrohyoid membrane is seen as an isoechoic line (hyperechoic air below) lying between hyoid bone and thyroid cartilage.[16]

ULTRASOUND GUIDANCE DURING PERCUTANEOUS DILATATIONAL TRACHEOSTOMY

Dreaded complications like bleeding, perforation of high mediastinal vessels, thyroid isthmus trauma, and stenosis of trachea can indeed be avoided, if ultrasound is used to identify the structures accurately.[17,18]

Structures within the lumen of the trachea or behind it are not seen very clearly, but very useful information can be obtained about pre or paratracheal structures.

Kollig et al. observed that nearly 25% of patients needed a change in the puncture site during the percutaneous procedure after ultrasound evaluation of the same.[19]

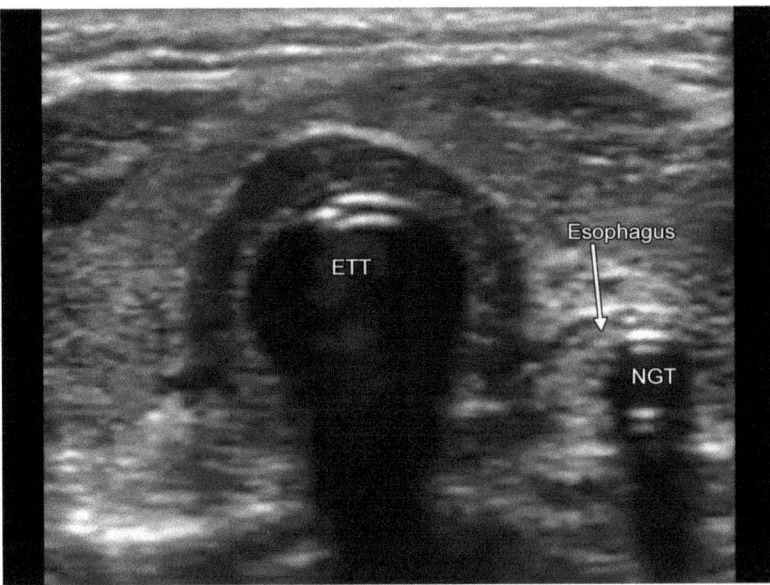

Fig. 3.7: Esophagus and nasogastric tube with endotracheal tube. (ETT: endotracheal tube; NGT; nasogastric tube)

The increased safety and success rate of ultrasonography (USG) guided percutaneous tracheostomy (PCT) has been reported in numerous studies.[18,20-22] Benefits of bedside ultrasound during the tracheostomy has also been demonstrated in morbidly obese patients with the BMI more than 34.[23]

Better success rates and faster time to successful cannulation have been observed by use of ultrasound compared to standard landmark method.[24]

In the traditional landmark versus ultrasound-guided evaluation trial (TARGET) study,[25] and one by Dinh et al.[26] it was observed that real-time ultrasound-guided attempts improve the success rate of percutaneous tracheotomy (PCT) at the first go with an improved accuracy for puncture site, as compared to traditional anatomical landmark methods being used.

Gobatto et al. observed during the Ultrasound Guided Percutaneous Tracheostomy versus Bronchoscopy Guided Percutaneous Tracheostomy (TRACHUS) randomized controlled trial, in critically ill patients, comparing POCUS-guided PCT with bronchoscopy-guided PCT, and concluded that POCUS-guided PCT was as good as bronchoscopy-guided PCT with regards to success rate and complications.[27]

Percutaneous Cricothyroidotomy with Ultrasound Guidance

Cricothyroidotomy, in an emergency, is life-saving in the "cannot intubate cannot ventilate" situation, but sometimes problems arise because the CTM is not easily identified by digital palpation guided by landmark techniques.[28,29]

Nicholls et al. identified the CTM with ultrasound guidance and proved its usefulness in its identification in their study. Visualization of the CTM was achieved in less than 25 sec with a rapid but shallow learning curve.[30] Curtis et al. also demonstrated identification of the CTM in less than 4 sec and completion of the procedure (USG-guided cricothyroidotomy) thus demonstrating a high success rate.[31] Siddiqui et al. demonstrated 3 time lower injury rate in ultrasound-guided procedures as compared to manual palpation and procedure method.[32]

Prediction and Evaluation of Postextubation Stridor

Measurement of the air column width at the level of the vocal cords by ultrasound and can potentially predict patients of postextubation stridor.

Ding et al.[33] studied the amount of air passing through the cords by comparing the air column width both before and after ETT cuff deflation. The chances of postextubation stridor were higher, if the change in air column width was less. Sutherasan et al.[34] observed mean air column width differences in patients with and without postextubation stridor is 1.99 mm and 1.08 mm, respectively, and observed a cutoff value of 1.6 mm as reasonably accurate in the prediction of postextubation stridor (sensitivity 70% and specificity of 70%) (negative predictive value—92% and positive predictive value—32%).

However, more studies with larger sample size are required to ascertain more accurately these cutoff points to help predict cases of postextubation stridor.

ASSESSMENT OF STOMACH

Sometimes, patients in emergencies may be at an increased risk of aspiration, or may require emergency surgical procedures, hence assessment of the stomach and gastric residue may also be quite important while assessing the airway in such patients.

CONCLUSION

Ultrasound for the upper airway assessment has much value in the critically ill patient.

It is portable, less invasive, cost effective, and can be reproduced multiple time at the point of care. Huge potential exists for the use and indeed incorporation into guidelines of upper airway ultrasound for the future.

REFERENCES

1. Adi O, Chuan TW, Rishya M. A feasibility study on bedside upper airway ultrasonography compared to waveform capnography for verifying endotracheal tube location after intubation. Crit Ultrasound J. 2013;5(1):7.
2. Chou EH, Dickman E, Tsou PY, et al. Ultrasonography for confirmation of endotracheal tube placement: a systematic review and meta-analysis. Resuscitation. 2015;90:97-103.
3. Shibasaki M, Nakajima Y, Ishii S, et al. Prediction of pediatric endotracheal tube size by ultrasonography. Anesthesiology. 2010;113(4):819-24.

4. Bae JY, Byon HJ, Han SS, et al. Usefulness of ultrasound for selecting a correctly sized uncuffed tracheal tube for paediatric patients. Anaesthesia. 2011;66(11):994-8.
5. Kim EJ, Kim SY, Kim WO, et al. Ultrasound measurement of subglottic diameter and an empirical formula for proper endotracheal tube fitting in children. Acta Anaesthesiol Scand. 2013;57(9):1124-30.
6. Lakhal K, Delplace X, Cottier JP, et al. The feasibility of ultrasound to assess subglottic diameter. Anesth Analg. 2007;104(3):611-4.
7. Sustic A, Miletic D, Protic A, et al. Can ultrasound be useful for predicting the size of a left double-lumen bronchial tube? Tracheal width as measured by ultrasonography versus computed tomography. J Clin Anesth. 2008;20(4):247-52.
8. Hui CM, Tsui BC. Sublingual ultrasound as an assessment method for predicting difficult intubation: a pilot study. Anaesthesia. 2014;69(4): 314-9.
9. Ezri T, Gewurtz G, Sessler DI, et al. Prediction of difficult laryngoscopy in obese patients by ultrasound quantification of anterior neck soft tissue. Anaesthesia. 2003;58:1111-4.
10. Adhikari S, Zeger W, Schmier C, et al. Pilot study to determine the utility of point-of-care ultrasound in the assessment of difficult laryngoscopy. Acad Emerg Med. 2011;18:754-58.
11. Marciniak B, Fayoux P, Hébrard A, et al. Airway management in children: Ultrasonography assessment of tracheal intubation in real time? Anesth Analg. 2009;108:461-5.
12. Sustic A. Role of ultrasound in the airway management of critically ill patients. Crit Care Med. 2007;3:173-7.
13. Das SK, Choupoo NS, Haldar R, et al. Transtracheal ultrasound for verification of endotracheal tube placement: a systematic review and meta-analysis. Can J Anaesth. 2015;62(4):413-23.
14. Chenkin J, McCartney CJ, Jelic T, et al. Defining the learning curve of point-of-care ultrasound for confirming endotracheal tube placement by emergency physicians. Crit Ultrasound J. 2015;7(1):14.
15. Chou EH, Dickman E, Tsou PY, et al. Ultrasonography for confirmation of endotracheal tube placement: a systematic review and meta-analysis. Resuscitation. 2015;90:97-103.
16. Green JS, Tsui BC. Applications of ultrasonography in ENT: Airway assessment and nerve blockade. Anesthesiol Clin. 2010;28:541-53.
17. Hatfield A, Bodenham A. Portable ultrasonic scanning of the anterior neck before percutaneous dilatational tracheostomy. Anaesthesia. 1999;54:660-3.
18. Sustić A, Kovac D, Zgaljardić Z, et al. Ultrasound-guided percutaneous dilatational tracheostomy: A safe method to avoid cranial misplacement of the tracheostomy tube. Intensive Care Med. 2000;26:1379-81.
19. Kollig E, Heydenreich U, Roetman B, et al. Ultrasound and bronchoscopic controlled percutaneous tracheostomy on trauma ICU. Injury. 2000;31(9):663-8.
20. Rajajee V, Fletcher JJ, Rochlen LR, et al. Real-time ultrasound-guided percutaneous dilatational tracheostomy: A feasibility study. Crit Care. 2011;15:R67.
21. Mitra S, Kapoor D, Srivastava M, et al. Ultrasound guided PDT in ICU. Indian J Crit Care Med. 2013;17:367-9.
22. Mehta Y. Percutaneous dilatational tracheostomy: Guided well with real-time ultrasound. Indian J Crit Care Med. 2013;17(6):335-6.
23. Guinot P, Zogheib E, Petiot S, et al. Ultrasound-guided percutaneous tracheostomy in critically ill obese patients. Critical Care. 2012;16:R40.
24. Dinsmore J, Heard AM, Green RJ. The use of ultrasound to guide time critical cannula tracheotomy when anterior neck airway anatomy is unidentifiable. Eur J Anaesthesiol. 2011;28(7):506-10.
25. Rudas M, Seppelt I, Herkes R, et al. Traditional landmark versus ultrasound guided tracheal puncture during percutaneous dilatational tracheostomy in adult intensive care patients: a randomised controlled trial. Crit Care. 2014;18(5):514.

26. Dinh VA, Farshidpanah S, Lu S, et al. Real-time sonographically guided percutaneous dilatational tracheostomy using a long-axis approach compared to the landmark technique. J Ultrasound Med. 2014;33(8):1407-542.
27. Gobatto AL, Besen BA, Tierno PF, et al. Ultrasound-guided percutaneous dilational tracheostomy versus bronchoscopy-guided percutaneous dilational tracheostomy in critically ill patients (TRACHUS): a randomized noninferiority controlled trial. Intensive Care Med. 2016;42(3):342-51
28. Bair AE, Chima R. The inaccuracy of using landmark techniques for cricothyroid membrane identification: a comparison of three techniques. Acad Emerg Med. 2015;22(8):908-14.
29. Elliott DS, Baker PA, Scott MR, et al. Accuracy of surface landmark identification for cannula cricothyroidotomy. Anaesthesia. 2010;65(9):889-94.
30. Nicholls SE, Sweeney TW, Ferre RM, et al. Bedside sonography by emergency physicians for the rapid identification of landmarks relevant to cricothyrotomy. Am J Emerg Med. 2008;26(8):852-6.
31. Curtis K, Ahern M, Dawson M, et al. Ultrasound-guided, Bougie-assisted cricothyroidotomy: a description of a novel technique in cadaveric models. Acad Emerg Med. 2012;19(7):876-9.
32. Siddiqui N, Arzola C, Friedman Z, et al. Ultrasound improves cricothyrotomy success in cadavers with poorly defined neck anatomy: a randomized control trial. Anesthesiology. 2015;123(5):1033-4.
33. Ding LW, Wang HC, Wu HD, et al. Laryngeal ultrasound: a useful method in predicting post-extubation stridor. A pilot study. Eur Respir J. 2006;27(2):384-9.
34. Sutherasan Y, Theerawit P, Hongphanut T, et al. Predicting laryngeal edema in intubated patients by portable intensive care unit ultrasound. J Crit Care. 2013;28(5):675-80.

CHAPTER 4

Ultrasound of the Lung and Clinical Uses in Emergencies

Pradeep D'Costa

INTRODUCTION

Air was once considered the graveyard for the ultrasound machine as it was considered a very poor medium of propagation of the ultrasound waves.

The lungs were once considered the worst enemy of the ultrasound machine and old editions of famous medicine textbooks (Harrison's Principles of Internal Medicine) have also commented on the possible futility of lung ultrasound to help clinical decision making.

But over the last three decades or so, substantial progress has been made in the field of lung ultrasound and this has indeed changed the approach toward the same in a very substantial manner.

Various protocols have been described bedside lung ultrasound in emergency (BLUE), fluid administration limited by lung sonography (FALLS), which have made the approach to a previously considered complex topic a very simplified one!

The whole of interpretation of the lung ultrasound is based on production and identification of various lung artifacts and their interpretation in the clinical scenario.

Professor Daniel Lichteinstein, by his pioneering work in this field from the 80s, has forever changed the way people look at the lungs with the ultrasound probe!!

BASIC INFORMATION

The whole of the lung ultrasound is based on two important principles:
1. Lungs are composed of mainly air.
2. Pathologies of the lung mostly involve changing this milieu of air to one composed predominantly of fluid, air, etc.

It is the interaction of the ultrasound beam with this air-fluid interface, which produces the typical artifacts based on which reasonably accurate diagnosis can be made.

This interaction produces many true and false images (artifacts) which can then be used to make important clinical decisions.

What follows is a short description of various artifacts that have been described.

Probe Positions (Fig. 4.1)

Various approaches have been described for performing lung ultrasound, but a basic layout has been described.

This involves examination of both lungs in various segments or intercostal spaces.

Each lung is commonly divided into around six various sections and each segment at least three intercostal spaces are scanned before ruling out or ruling in any pathology.

Commonly each lung is divided into six segments as shown in the diagram by anterior and posterior axillary lines (Figs. 4.1).

Probes Used

Commonly used probes (Fig. 4.2A and B) for lung ultrasound include:
- Linear probe—higher frequency—commonly to study the superficial layers like pleura and superficial lung surfaces
- Convex probe—medium-frequency probe—commonly used to study the deeper structures of the lung better.

Normal Appearances

A Normal Lung

Appearances of normal pleura:
- The normal pleura, composed of the parietal and visceral layers, is seen on the ultrasound image as a thick white, homogenous line.

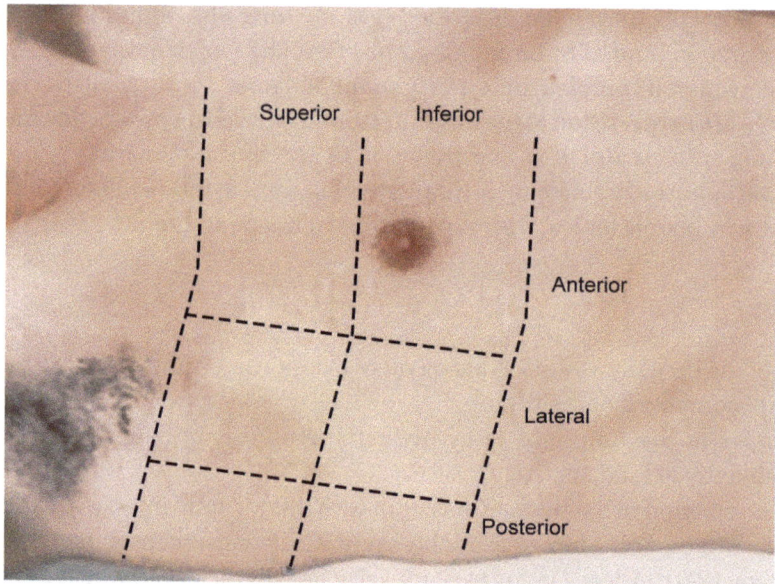

Fig. 4.1: Probe positions.

Ultrasound of the Lung and Clinical Uses in Emergencies 33

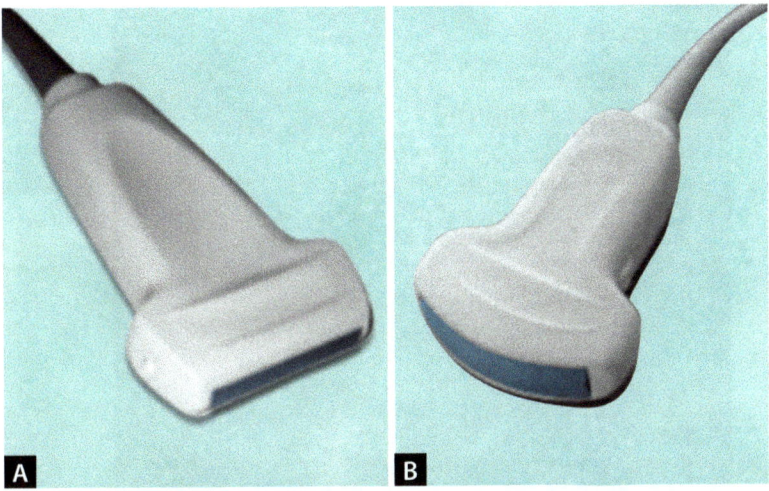

Figs. 4.2A and B: Various probes used for lung ultrasound.

- Due to the dynamic nature of lung expansion with each breath, the pleura are seen to move in a horizontal manner with each respiration, this is called "the pleural sliding sign".
- It indicates a mobile lung.

Pathologies:
- Thickening of the pleura, immobility of the pleura, or reduced mobility of the pleura have been described.
- A pleural slide indicates a mobile lung under the pleura.

Normal lung profile
A normal lung segment is one in which you see:
- Normal lung sliding or pleural sliding
- Horizontal reverberation artifacts—the *"A" lines.*

The "A" line:
- When the ultrasound probe is placed on the chest wall, the structures encountered by the beam include skin, subcutaneous tissue, intercostal muscles, nerves, and then the pleura.
- Once, the ultrasound beam reaches the pleura, it bounces back to the probe and reappears on the screen as a white horizontal line, which is equidistant as the pleural line.
- This white horizontal line is a "reverberation" artifact and is called the A line.
- Subsequent images on the screen produce multiple such horizontal lines, the further from the screen the more faint would be the line.
- This A profile along with the pleural sliding sign indicates a normally mobile lung.

Upon M-mode imaging through this lung segment we would get an image which would look like the seashore (i.e. immobile skin, subcut tissue, and muscles—these are the true images and give the appearance of "sea", and a dynamically moving lung beneath producing the granular appearance—shore, these are the false images), leading to this appearance being described as "the seashore sign" (Figs. 4.3A to C).

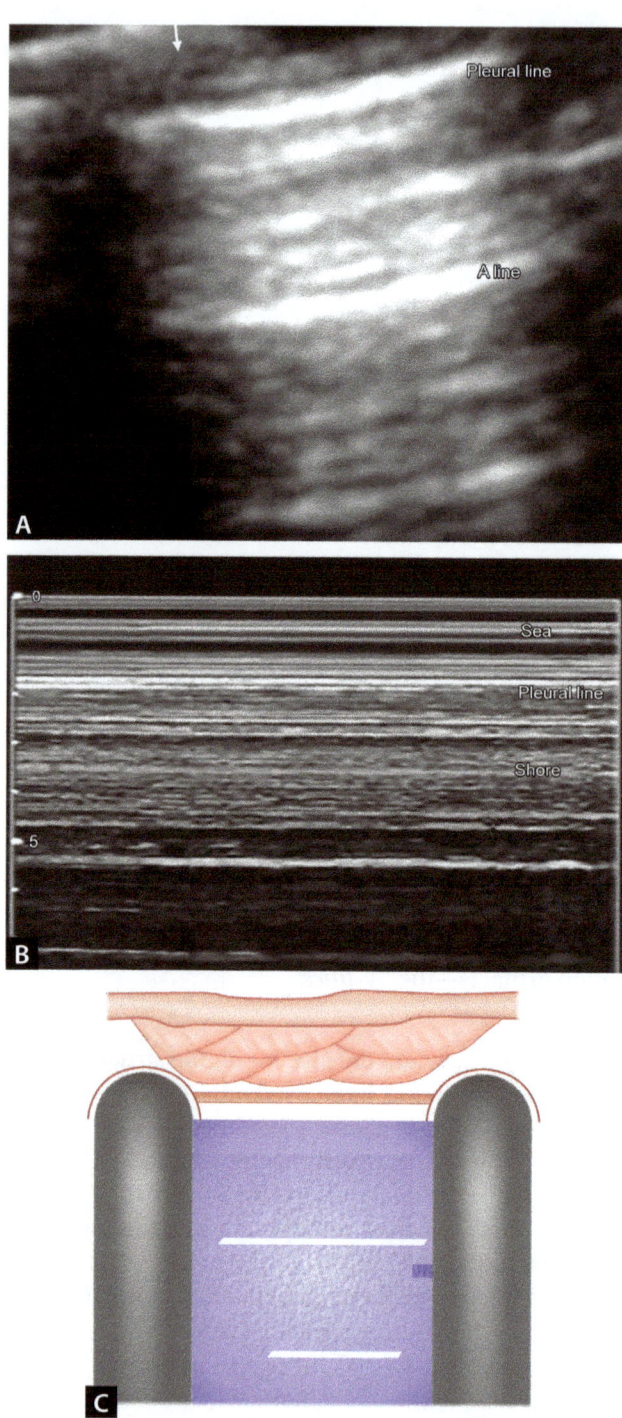

Figs. 4.3A to C: (A) A profile; (B) Seashore sign; (C) Anatomy of normal lung.

While a "wet" lung can be identified by the following characteristics.

B lines:
- These are vertical lines starting from the subpleural area
- Traverse the whole ultrasound screen
- They abolish the A lines
- They are thick and white lines
- They usually indicate fluid in the alveolar interstitial space
- Previous nomenclature called these lines included terms like "lung comets" or "lung rockets"
- The severity of the fluid-filled lungs was previously interpreted by measuring the amount or distance between two B lines
- Hence, the terms B3 or B7 lung rockets were introduced
- Hence, B3 rockets meant much more fluid-filled lungs than B 7 rockets (Figs. 4.4A to C).

The Z line:
- Many a times, vertical lines appear on the screen which may mimic B lines.
- The difference between the B lines and Z lines are that the Z lines do not traverse to the end of the screen, and they do not erase the A lines.
- These lines are a normal variant and do not signify anything abnormal.

The E lines:
- These lines are also called "emphysema" lines.
- They are commonly seen when there is subcutaneous tissue air.
- What differentiates these lines from the "B" lines is the origin of the line, much higher than pleural line and the masking of all other architecture based on the fact that air is a very poor conductor of the ultrasound beam.
- These lines are commonly seen in patients of subcutaneous emphysema.

Now, the lung is studied in various segments both anteriorly and posteriorly, bilaterally to avoid missing any pathology.

Many typical profiles can give invaluable clues to the diagnosis of the underlying pathology and hence make treatment decisions easier.
- Bilateral symmetrical B lines, many times more at bases than at the apices and many times associated with a 2D ECHO finding of a low systolic function or evidence of diastolic dysfunction make the possibility of cardiogenic pulmonary edema more likely.
- Bilateral lung fields showing a varied and different appearance, e.g. (A) profile in a segment, (B) in the adjoining segment, and (C) a profile (consolidation type) in certain segments point more in favor of a noncardiac cause of the problem like acute respiratory distress syndrome (ARDS), pneumonia, lung contusion, etc.
    - *The C profile or consolidation features:*
        - Typical identification of lung infective foci can also be accurately diagnosed by the use of bedside ultrasound.
        - The lung exhibits the following patterns of consolidation.
        - The initial stage development of small subpleural consolidations, this is the stage of microconsolidation.

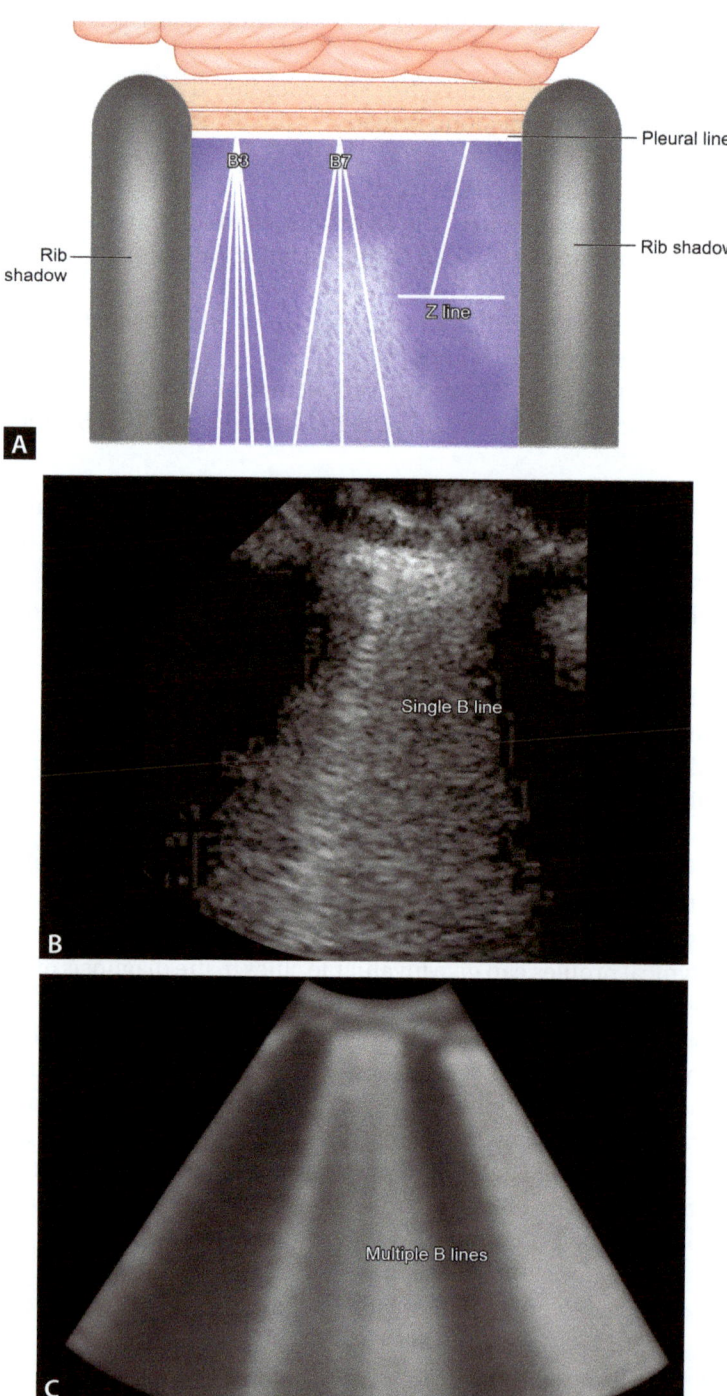

Figs. 4.4A to C: (A) Wet lung profiles, B-lines or B3 or B7-lines; (B) Single B-line; (C) Multiple B-lines.

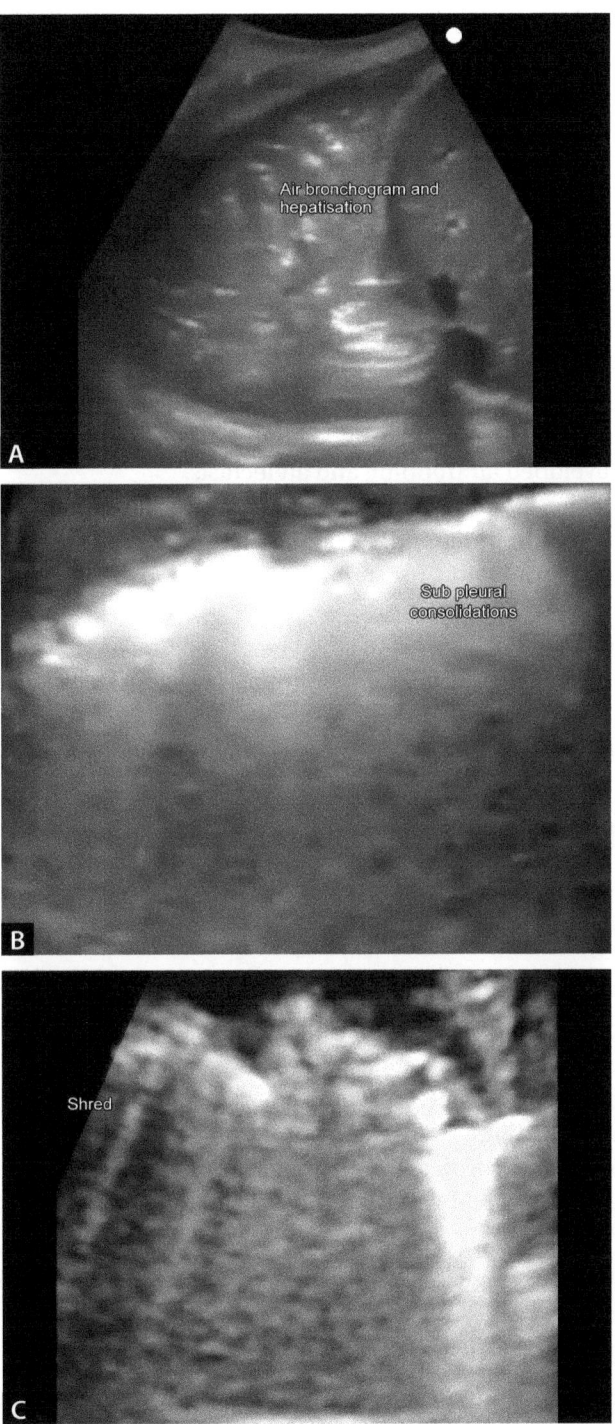

Figs. 4.5A to C: (A) Air bronchogram (note white dots); (B) Subpleural consolidations; (C) SHRED sign—note multiple irregular "B" lines from multiple levels with surrounding pleural effusion.

- As more lung areas start getting involved, macroconsolidation like changes set in and involve larger lung areas.
- These areas exhibit some "wet" lung profiles, but in addition may exhibit the "shred" sign—appearance of an irregular distorted pleural line, with appearance of B lines arising from various levels.
- The tissue like sign—the lung parenchyma on the ultrasound looks exactly like a solid organ, commonly compared to the liver and spleen. This has been described in pathology textbooks as the stage of "hepatization" of lung parenchyma.
- The air bronchogram—the appearance of air moving in and out of the terminal airways can be well picked up by the ultrasound, and gives the appearance of white dots moving dynamically with respiration—this has been described as a "true consolidation pattern" or a dynamic air bronchogram (Figs. 4.5A to C).
- A static air bronchogram, on the other hand, could imply areas of the lung, which have developed air trapping and atelectasis.
- The *"lung pulse"* on the other hand, many a times is confused with "lung point", but is a totally independent sign, is a typical finding of the cardiac pulsations being transmitted to a nonaerated lungs, and giving the appearance of a pulsating lung.
- The causes of the lung pulse could be of a significant nature (e.g. lung collapse due to a unilateral lung intubation or mucus plug block of a bronchus).

– *Diagnosis of a pneumothorax by ultrasound:*
We will look at the lungs, inferior vena cava (IVC) for making a diagnosis.

LUNG FINDINGS IN PNEUMOTHORAX (FIGS. 4.6A TO C)

The following diagnostic criteria are usually present in a case of a pneumothorax:
- Absence of lung sliding
- A profile
- Presence of B profile, C profile, lung sliding, and lung pulse effectively rules out a pneumothorax in the lung segment studied
- Presence of stratosphere or barcode sign—this is the appearance of the lung on M mode, which is immobile and may be present in a patient who has a pneumothorax
- Presence of the "lung point"—this is the point on the chest wall where during inspiration, the lung expands and creates a typical seashore sign on M mode, and on expiration there is only air present beneath the probe giving the typical "barcode" or "stratosphere" sign.

This lung point when found is the most accurate sign of the presence of a pneumothorax.

Inferior Vena Cava

- The IVC—many times a dilated and turgid IVC is encountered in these patients.
- Heart—unless a coexisting cardiac pathology, the systolic cardiac function is normal.

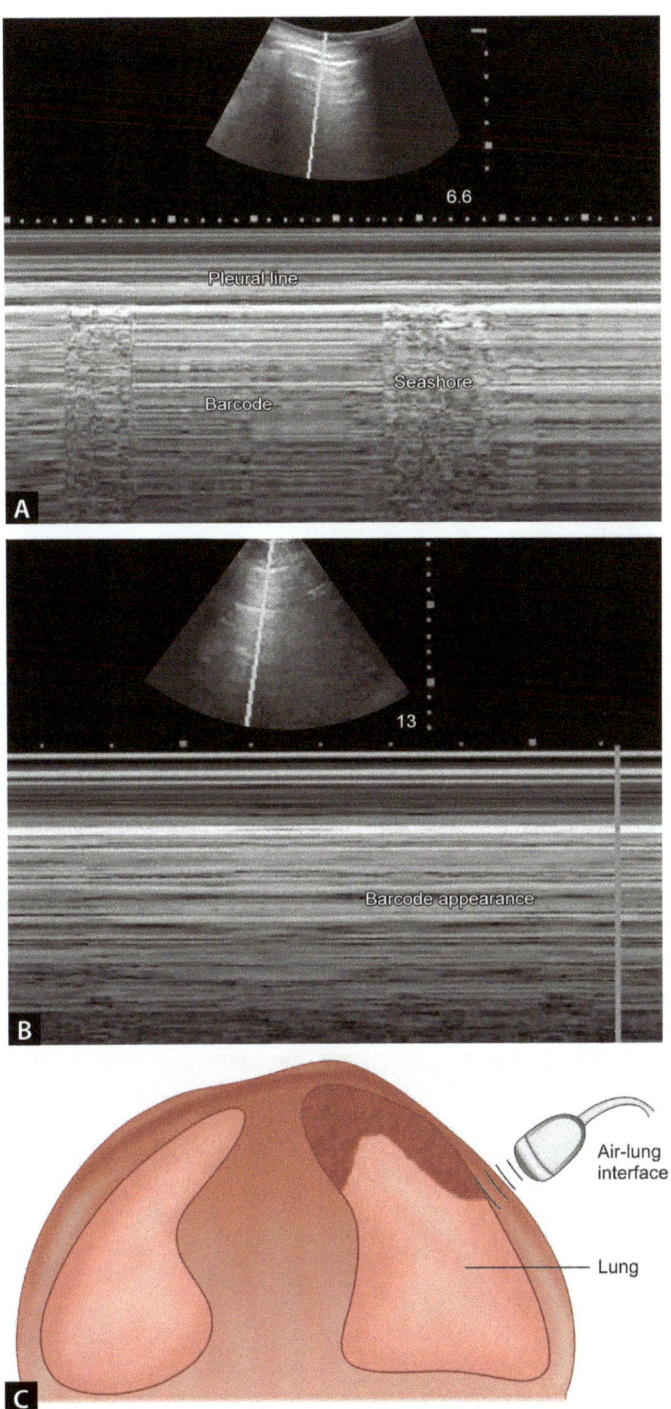

Figs. 4.6A to C: (A) The lung point; (B) Barcode or stratosphere sign, and lung point (note barcode alternating with seashore sign); (C) Pneumothorax—location of lung point.

PLEURAL EFFUSION (FIGS. 4.7A TO D)

- A pleural effusion is usually diagnosed as an echo-free area seen between the visceral and parietal pleura.
- Contours of the effusion vary with different phases of respiration and also with the posture of the patient.
- Pleural effusions are also identified by the sinusoid or quad sign.
- When an M-mode image is taken through the area of interest, the effusion gives a typical appearance of a "sinusoid" or a "quad".
- The pleural effusion is delineated by the following borders—(1) the pleural line, (2 and 3) the shadow of the ribs, and (4) the lung line (visceral pleura), this has been described as the *quad sign*.
  – It is a static sign.
- On application of M-mode, real-time images show the lung line moving toward the pleural line on inspiration. This has been described as *sinusoid sign*.
  – It is a dynamic sign

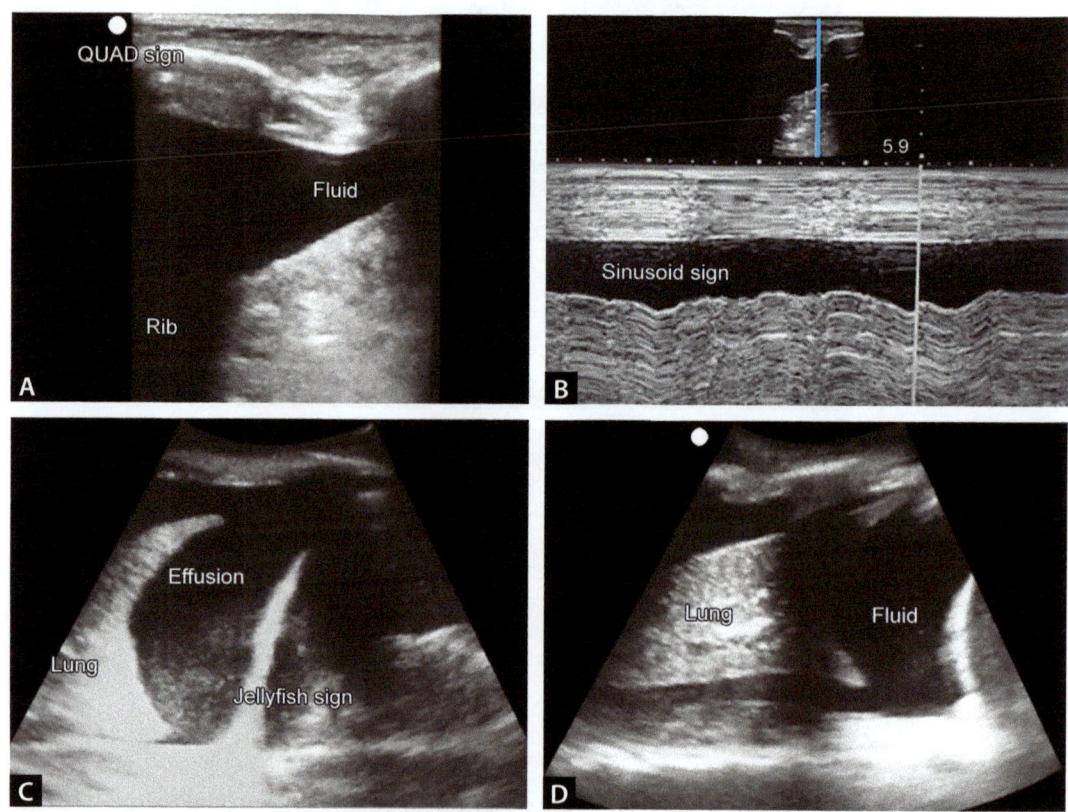

Figs. 4.7A to D: The sonographic appearance of pleural effusion.

- The jellyfish sign
  - The sight of a freely moving lung within free fluid gives the appearance of a jellyfish moving in water and hence has been described as some as the jellyfish sign.

The sonographic appearance of pleural effusion depends on the cause, nature, and duration of the collection.

Different appearances that may be observed include:
- Anechoic—usually clear and featureless
- Transudates are mostly anechoic
- Complex but nonseptated
- Complex and septated
- Echogenic
- Complex, septated, and echogenic fluid is usually exudative in nature
- Inflammatory effusions commonly produce strands.
- The clinical relevance to knowing the type of effusion is that thoracocentesis is usually possible in effusions that are anechoic, complex, or complex with movable septae
- Sometimes confusion may exist in between a pleural thickening and an effusion.

Types of Effusions (Figs. 4.8A to C)

- Septate effusion
- The *"fluid color sign"*
- Transmitted respiratory and/or cardiac pulsations may exhibit a signal in a case of effusion and are absent in pleural thickening
- This fact may be useful when the effusion is of a very small quantity (sensitivity 89.2, specificity 100%)
- Thoracocentesis
- *Safe puncture:* More than three intercostal spaces with in-plane (IP) distance more than 1.5 cm; absence of interposition of lung, heart, liver, and spleen; interpleural distance variation; and mark best puncture point and fixed patient position. (0% complications).

DIAPHRAGM (FIGS. 4.9A AND B)

- The utility of ultrasound in diaphragm movements has been taken advantage of in various studies.
- Movements of the diaphragm have been studied during weaning trials and have found a good correlation with weaning.
- Identified by its deep location, curved geometry, and muscular echotexture.
- Longitudinally, muscles have a mixed echogenic appearance, consisting of hypoechoic (dark) muscle fibers separated by hyperechoic (bright) fibroadipose septae (perimysium).
- Transversely, the mixed echogenicity pattern of muscle produces a "starry night" appearance.
- The diaphragm can be seen as 2 echogenic layers of peritoneum and pleura sandwiching a more hypoechoic line of the muscle itself (Fig. 4.10).

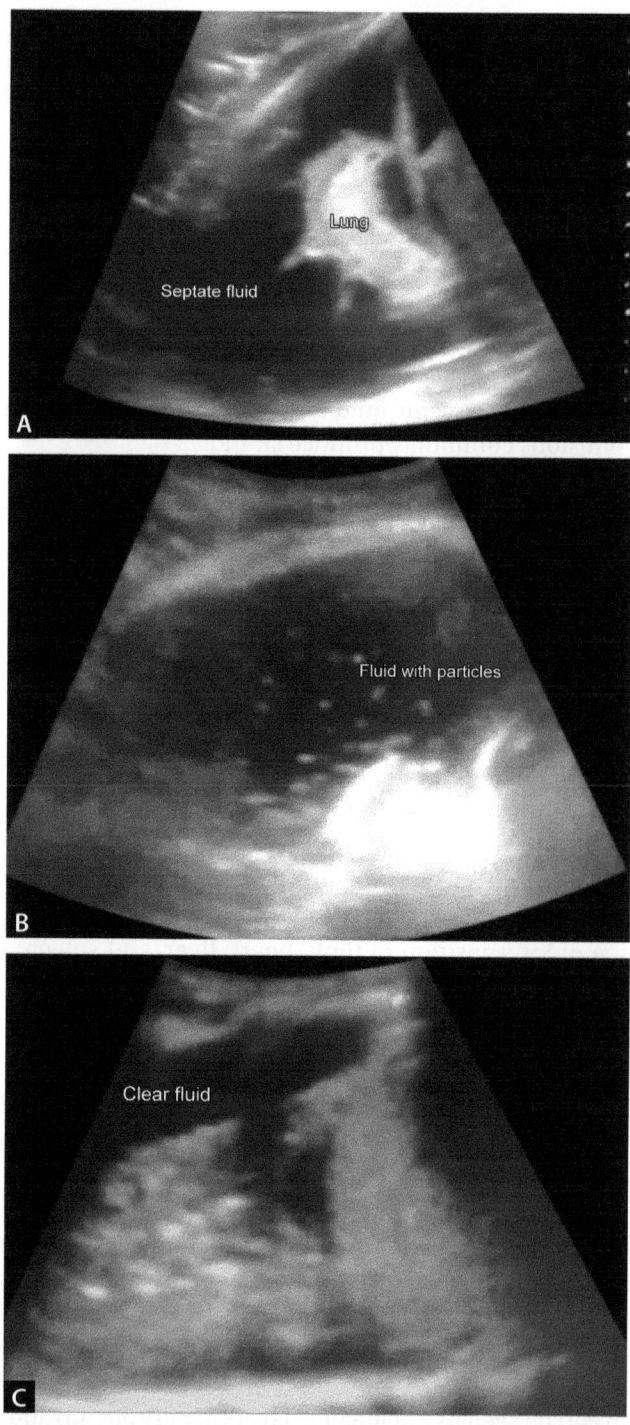

Figs. 4.8A to C: (A) Exudative effusion with fibrin strands; (B) Pleural fluid with particulate matter; (C) Transudative effusion-clear.

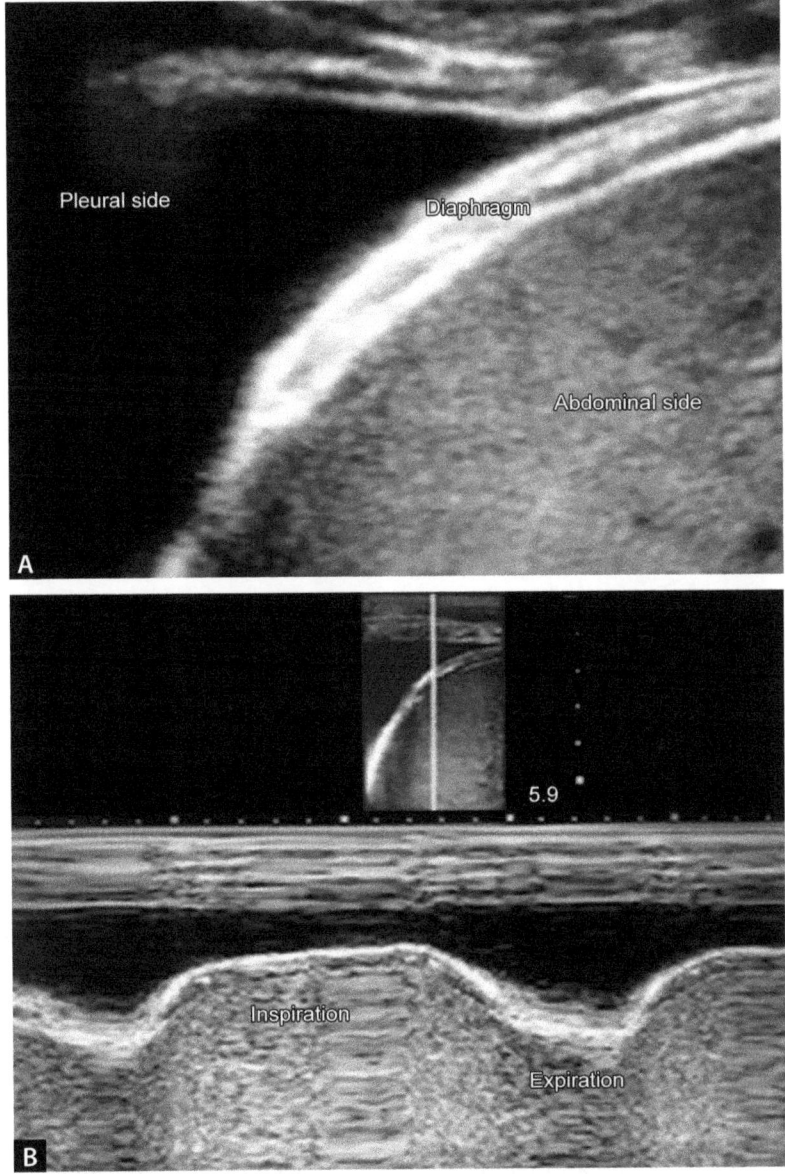

Figs. 4.9A and B: (A) Normal diaphragm anatomy; (B) Diaphragm movements.

- It thickens during inspiration, unless it is severely atrophic.
- An atrophic diaphragm will appear as a very thin strip deep to the intercostal muscles, and it may not move with inspiration
- Thickness and echogenicity of the diaphragm can be assessed using B mode ultrasound

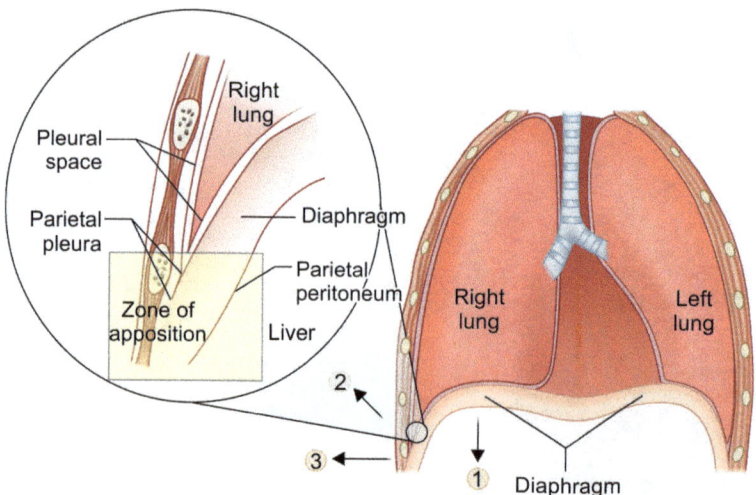

Figs. 4.10: Basic anatomy of diaphragm (1: intra abdominal; 2: lung; 3: diaphragm).

- M mode ultrasound, can assess excursion (including side-to-side variability), velocity, and response to phrenic nerve stimulation.
- The average thickness of the diaphragm is 0.22–0.28 cm in healthy volunteers and 0.13–0.19 cm in a paralyzed diaphragm.
- A diaphragm thickness less than 0.2 cm, measured at the end of expiration, has been proposed as the cut-off to define diaphragm atrophy.

LUNG ULTRASOUND USE IN THE CRITICAL CARE SETTING

- The critically ill patient on ventilator presents a whole lot of challenges to the treating clinician.
- A patient who is hypoxic requires an urgent trouble shooting to locate the cause of the problems, which may be lifesaving.
- Many times dilemmas exist in the mind of the treating physician—should I transfuse fluids? should I increase positive end-expiratory pressure (PEEP), and is a bronchoscopy indicated? why is there failure to ventilate properly? etc.
- The ultrasound can be an invaluable tool in this confusion and helps to answer many unanswered questions in case only X-rays are relied on.

The following are just some of the possible uses of the ultrasound in such a situation

Ultrasound use for the Management of the ARDS Patient

- Assessing the lungs in a patient who has severe lung injury has found new scope in the critically ill patients.
- Being noninvasive, it has definite additional benefits.

- The ultrasound can be used to:
  - Perform recruitment maneuvers—define opening and closing pressures. Tusman et al. have described a four stage assessment of the lung while performing recruitment maneuvers.
    - Step 1—assessment assess for lung collapse of deaeration
    - Step 2—assess the clinical condition and likelihood of tolerating a maneuver
    - Step 3—determine the lungs opening pressures, i.e. the stage at which the deaeration picture changes to a reaeration one (consolidation or B profile to A profile)
    - Step 4—determining the closing pressures. Stepwise reduction in PEEP is done till deaeration just begins. This is the closing pressure.

Positive end-expiratory pressure is then set at a level slightly higher than this pressure. This is the "open lung" pressure.

Assess the Extravascular Lung Water Component

Quite accurately—many times comparable with conventional methods like pulse index cardiac output (PiCO), etc. Zen Zhao et al. have also assessed the utility of the ultrasonography (USG) versus pulse index continuous cardiac output (PiCCO) and found good correlation between the two methods.

Diagnosing very Early a Ventilator-associated Pneumonia

Usually, a pneumonia is caused by air volume changes in the lungs. Various methods used to make a diagnosis of ventilator-associated pneumonia (VAP) include conventional radiographs (new shadows), or even by changes in fraction of inspired oxygen (FiO_2) and PEEP (quantitative and objective).

Some authors have also explored the use of a score which utilizes ultrasound, procalcitonin, and infection score, scores of more than 5 were found to be better in predicting a VAP than the clinical pulmonary infection score (CPIS).

In addition to making a diagnosis, it is also useful in monitoring the progress of a new "shadow".

Assessing the Effects of PEEP by Using a Lung Aeration or Deaeration Score

Components of this score include four ultrasound aeration patterns:
1. Normal aeration (N)
2. Moderate aeration loss—multiple well-defined "B" lines—B1
3. Severe aeration loss—multiple coalescent "B" lines—B2
4. Lung consolidation—C.

Accordingly quantification of reaeration was done by assigning following points (Table 4.1):

The quantification of loss of aeration was done by a similar score and points (Table 4.2):

Table 4.1: Quantification of reaeration.

1 point	3 points	5 points
B1 > N	B2 > N	C > N
B2 > B1	C > B1	
C > B2		

Table 4.2: Quantification of loss of aeration.

5 points	3 points	1 point
N > C	N > B2	N > B1
	B1 > C	B1 > B2
		B2 > C

- An ultrasound reaeration score of +8 or higher was associated with a PEEP-induced lung recruitment greater than 600 mL.
- An ultrasound lung reaeration score of + 4 or less was associated with a PEEP-induced lung recruitment ranging from 75 mL to 450 mL.

Differentiating Cardiogenic from Noncardiogenic Pulmonary Edema

Ultrasound features which are homogeneous in distribution, show relatively regular pleural outlines and may be associated with bilateral effusions (pleural) will favor a cardiogenic origin of course cardiac ultrasound would add weight to this diagnosis, while an inhomogeneous distribution, with some "sparing" of areas, with sometimes pleural irregularities and consolidations, varied lung signs go in favor of an ARDS pathology.

BEDSIDE LUNG ULTRASOUND IN EMERGENCY PROTOCOL (FLOWCHART 4.1)

- The BLUE protocol can be used for a breathless patient, who is admitted to the emergency unit.
- This protocol gives us a very simplified decision making tree to the possible etiology of the respiratory failure of the main causes of acute respiratory failure.
- The protocol claims to have an overall 90.5% accuracy.
- The BLUE protocol combines signs, location, and in seven profiles
- The A-profile associates anterior lung sliding with A-lines.
- The A'-profile is an A-profile with no lung sliding.
    - The B-profile associates anterior lung sliding with lung comets.
    - The B'-profile is a B-profile with absent lung sliding.
    - The C-profile indicates anterior lung consolidation.
    - The A or B profile, both profiles appearing in different lung areas.

Flowchart. 4.1: BLUE protocol.

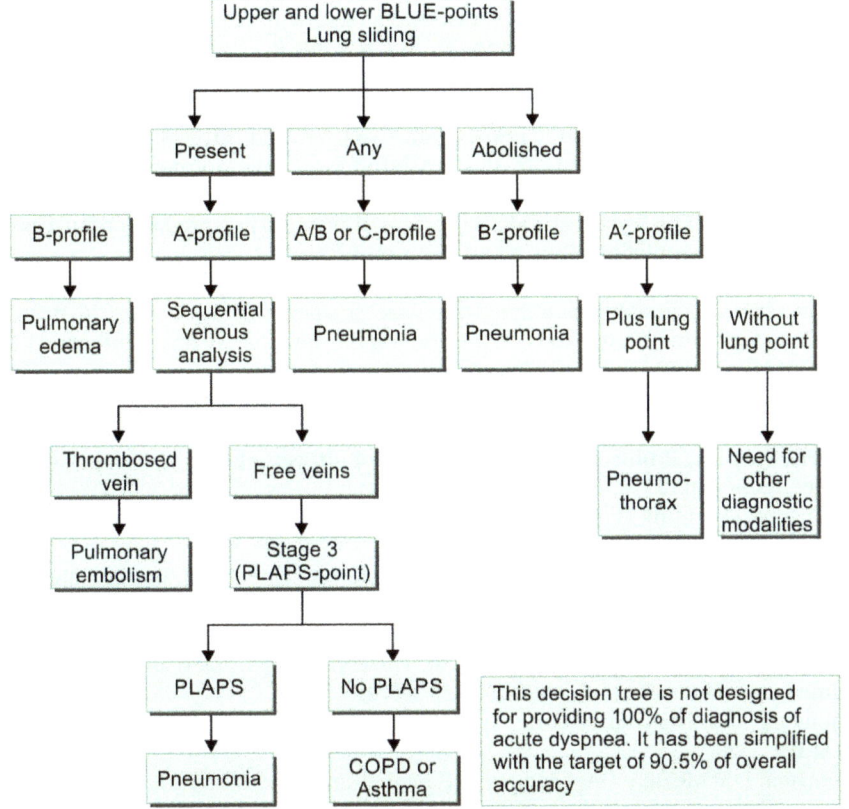

(BLUE: Bedside lung ultrasound in emergency; PLAPS: Posterolateral alveolar and/or pleural syndrome)

FLUID ADMINISTRATION LIMITED BY LUNG SONOGRAPHY PROTOCOL

The FALLS protocol have been published, showing the correlation between an A-profile or equivalents (A- or B-profile) and a low pulmonary artery occlusion pressure (PAOP), with a 18 mm Hg value occurring when B-lines appear

Hence, patients with the predominant profile of A are called "FALLS responders".

When the profile changes to a B predominant profile the end point of fluid resuscitation is reached.

CONCLUSION

- Lung ultrasound is an invaluable tool in the hands of the critical care physician.
- It helps take, modify, and do interventions at the bedside, which go a long way in making the care more accurate and tailor-made.
- Ultrasound will be the way forward for critical care!!

FURTHER READING

1. Ali ER, Mohamad AM. Diaphragm ultrasound as a new functional and morphological index of outcome, prognosis and discontinuation from mechanical ventilation in critically ill patients and evaluating the possible protective indices against VIDD. Egyptian J Chest Dis Tuberculo. 2017.
2. Bouhemad B, Liu ZH, Arbelot C, et al. Ultrasound assessment of antibiotic-induced pulmonary reaeration in ventilator-associated pneumonia. Crit Care Med. 2010;38:84-92.
3. Bouhemad B, Mongodi S, Via G, et al. Ultrasound for "Lung Monitoring" of Ventilated Patients. Anesthesiology. 2015;122:437-47.
4. DiNino E, Gartman EJ, Sethi JM, et al. Diaphragm ultrasound as a predictor of successful extubation from mechanical ventilation. Thorax. 2014;69:423-7.
5. Enghard P, Rademacher S, Nee J, et al. Simplified lung ultrasound protocol shows excellent prediction of extravascular lung water in ventilated intensive care patients. Crit Care. 2015;19:36.
6. Husain LF, Hagopian L, Wayman D, et al. Sonographic diagnosis of pneumothorax. J Emerg Trauma Shock. 2012;5(1):76-81.
7. Jiang JR, Tsai TH, Jerng JS, et al. Ultrasonographic evaluation of liver/spleen movements and extubation outcome. Chest. 2004;126:179-85.
8. Laing FC, Filly RA. Problems in the application of ultrasonography for the evaluation of pleural opacities. Radiology. 1978;126:211-4.
9. Lichteinstein DA. Lung Ultrasound in the Critically Ill-The BLUE Protocol. Switzerland: Springer International Publishing; 2016.
10. Lichteinstein DA. Whole body ultrasonography in the critically ill. Berlin Heidelberg: Springer-Verlag; 2010.
11. Lichtensteiin DA. General ultrasound in the critically ill. Berlin Heidelberg: Springer-Verlag; 2005.
12. Lichtenstein D, Meziere G, Biderman P, et al. The comet tail artifact: an ultrasound sign ruling out pneumothorax. Intensive Care Med. 1999;25:383-8.
13. Lichtenstein DA, Mauriat P. Lung Ultrasound in the Critically Ill Neonate. Curr Pediatr Rev. 2012;8(3):217-23.
14. Lichtenstein DA, Mezière GA, Lagoueyte JF, et al. A-lines and B-lines: lung ultrasound as a bedside tool for predicting pulmonary artery occlusion pressure in the critically ill. Chest. 2009;136:1014-20.
15. Lichtenstein DA. BLUE-protocol and FALLS-protocol: two applications of lung ultrasound in the critically ill. Chest. 2015;147(6):1659-70.
16. Lichtenstein DA. Lung ultrasound in the critically ill. Ann Intensive Care. 2014;4:1.
17. Mayo P, Volpicelli G, Lerolle N, et al. Ultrasonography evaluation during the weaning process: the heart, the diaphragm, the pleura and the lung. Intensive Care Med. 2016;42:1107-17.
18. Tusman G, Acosta CM, Nicola M, et al. Real-time images of tidal recruitment using lung ultrasound. Crit Ultrasound J. 2015;7:19.
19. Volpicelli G, Elbarbary M, Blaivas M, et al. International evidence-based recommendations for point-of-care lung ultrasound. Intensive Care Med. 2012;38(4):577-91.
20. Wang G, Ji X, Xu Y, et al. Lung ultrasound: a promising tool to monitor ventilator-associated pneumonia in critically ill patients. Crit Care. 2016;20:320.
21. Wu RG, Yang PC, Kuo SH, et al. "Fluid color" sign: a useful indicator for discrimination between pleural thickening and pleural effusion. J Ultrasound Med. 1995;14:767-9.
22. Yang PC, Luh KT, Chang DB, et al. Value of sonography in determining the nature of pleural effusion: analysis of 320 cases. AJR Am J Roentgenol. 1992;159:29-33.
23. Zagli G, Cozzolino M, Terreni A, et al. Diagnosis of ventilator-associated pneumonia: a pilot, exploratory analysis of a new score based on procalcitonin and chest echography. Chest. 2014;146(6):1578-85.
24. Zhao Z, Jiang L, Xi X, et al. Prognostic value of extravascular lung water assessed with lung ultrasound score by chest sonography in patients with acute respiratory distress syndrome. BMC Pulmonary Med. 2015;15:98.

CHAPTER 5

Focused Cardiac Ultrasound

J Chacko, Jayant Shelgaonkar, Rahul Pandit, Charudutt Vaity

Part 1: Focused Cardiac Ultrasound for the Acute Care Physician— Basic Views, Anatomy, and Measurements

J Chacko

BASIC ECHOCARDIOGRAPHIC VIEWS

Transducer position for basic echocardiographic views is depicted in Figure 5.1.

Apical 4-chamber View

For the apical 4-chamber (A4C) view, the patient ideally lies in the left lateral position. However, in many critically ill patients, it may not be easy to reposition the patient, especially if repeated examinations are required. In most patients, a supine position may offer adequate views. The transducer is placed at the point of the apex beat, usually in the fourth or the fifth intercostal space, with the probe marker pointing to the left shoulder. By manipulating the transducer from side to side and from one intercostal space to the other, optimal views are obtained (Fig. 5.2).

In the A4C view, all the four chambers are assessed, and the left ventricular (LV) systolic function and wall motion abnormalities are evaluated. The LV size and presence of hypertrophy may be readily identified. The right heart size and function are also assessed on this view. The function of the mitral and tricuspid valves is also evaluated.

Apical 5-chamber View

The apical 5-chamber (A5C) view is obtained by gradually tilting the probe downwards from the A4C position (Fig. 5.3). On this view, in addition to the atria and the ventricles, the LV outflow tract (LVOT) and the aortic valve (AV) are seen. Pulse wave (PW) Doppler of the LVOT is used to measure stroke volume (SV).

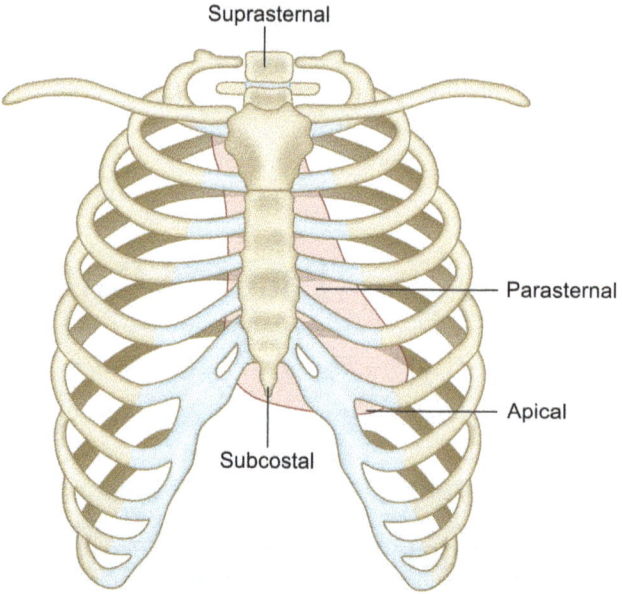

Fig. 5.1: Transducer position for basic echocardiographic views.

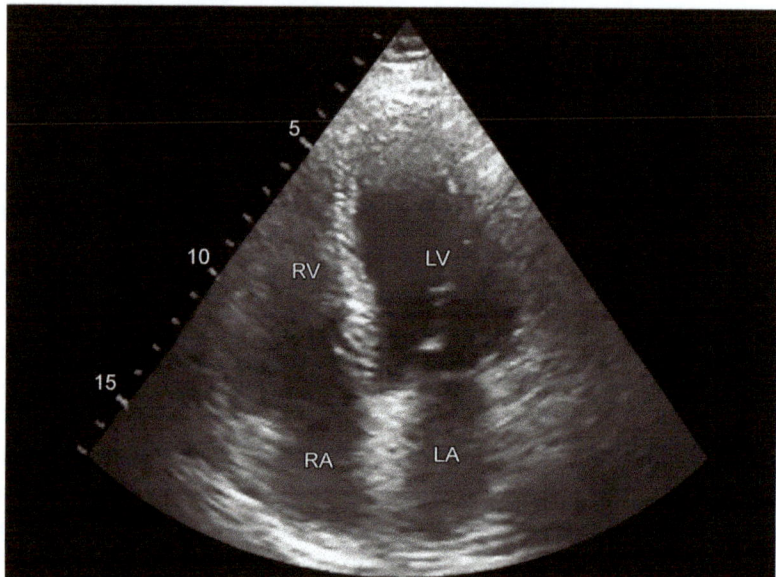

Fig. 5.2: The apical 4-chamber view.
(LA: left atrium; LV: left ventricular; RA: right atrium; RV: right ventricular)

Parasternal Long-axis View

The parasternal long-axis (PLAX) view (Fig. 5.4) is obtained by placing the transducer on the left parasternal border in the second or the third intercostal space; and the probe marker

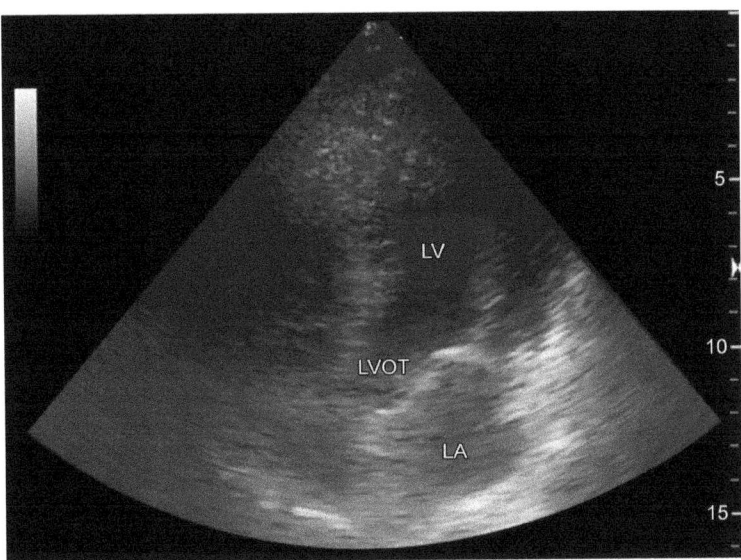

Fig. 5.3: The apical 5-chamber view.
(LA: left atrium; LV: left ventricular; LVOT: left ventricular outflow tract)

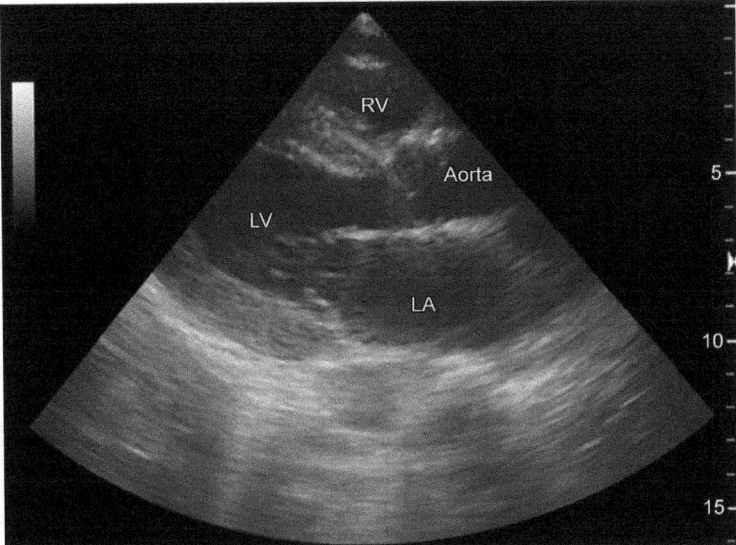

Fig. 5.4: The parasternal long axis view.
(LA: left atrium; LV: left ventricular; RV: right ventricular)

points to the right shoulder of the patient. On this view, the LV and the left atrium (LA) are seen toward the bottom of image; and the right ventricle (RV) is seen above the LV. The LVOT and the AV are also visualized on the PLAX view. Aortic and mitral valve (MV) function, size of the ventricles and the LA, and the LV function are assessed on this view.

Parasternal Short-axis View

To obtain the parasternal short-axis (PSAX) view, the transducer is rotated gradually in a clockwise direction from the PLAX view till the probe marker points cranially. By manipulation and repositioning, a view, as in Figure 5.5, is obtained. On the PSAX view, both ventricles are visualized in the cross-sectional view. The LV may be viewed at several levels, including the MV and the papillary muscles. The PSAX view offers information regarding size and function of both ventricles, anatomy and function of the MV, and presence of pericardial collection.

Subcostal View

In many critically ill patients who are on mechanical ventilation, echocardiographic views may be affected by lung inflation that may obscure conventional windows. This is more pronounced, if high-ventilation pressures are being used. In this situation, it may be possible to obtain a reasonably good view of the heart from the subcostal view. The transducer is placed just below the xiphoid process with the probe marker pointing to the left of the patient. An echocardiographic view similar to the A4C is obtained (Fig. 5.6). The subcostal view offers similar information to the A4C in a mechanically ventilated patient with limited windows.

INFERIOR VENA CAVA

The inferior vena cava (IVC) is commonly viewed from the epigastric region. A low-frequency transducer (3–5 MHz) is placed just below the sternum in the horizontal axis. This enables

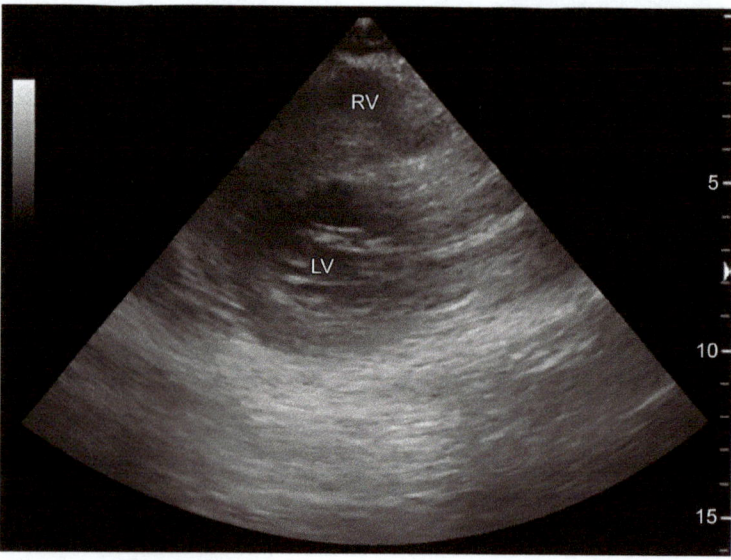

Fig. 5.5: The parasternal short-axis view.
(LV: left ventricular; RV: right ventricular)

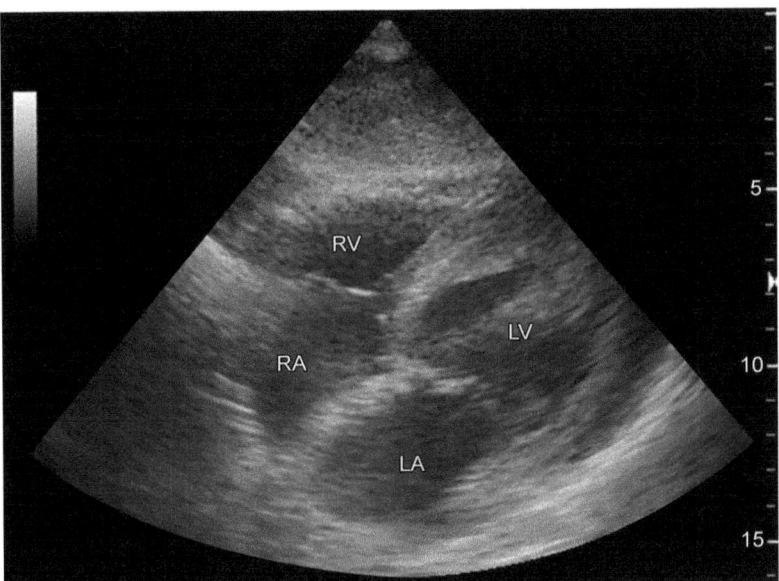

Fig. 5.6: The subcostal view.
(LA: left atrium; LV: left ventricular; RA: right atrium; RV: right ventricular)

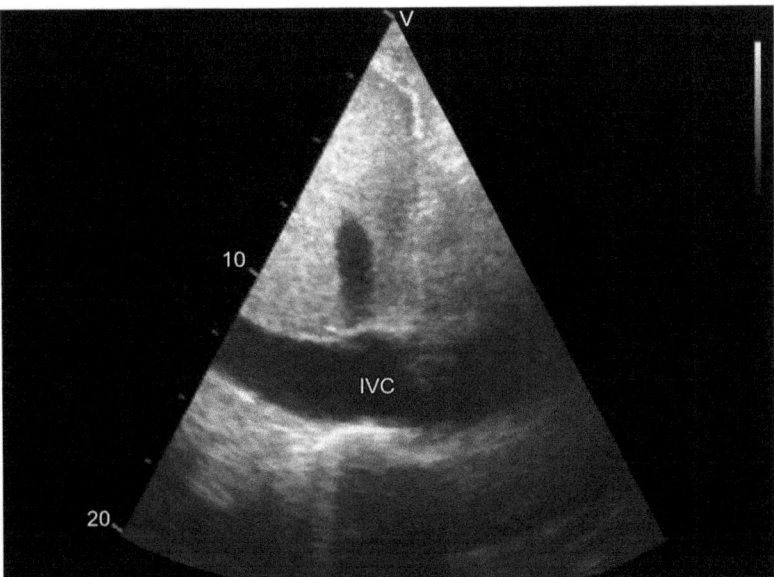

Fig. 5.7: The long-axis view of the inferior vena cava (IVC).

visualization of the IVC and the aorta in the short axis. The next step is to turn the probe clockwise with the probe marker directed to the head of the patient. This IVC is now seen in its long axis (Fig. 5.7). Measurements are made after switching to the M-mode view.

ASSESSMENT OF VOLUME RESPONSIVENESS USING ULTRASONOGRAPHY

Conventional indicators of preload assessment including the central venous pressure and the pulmonary capillary pressure are poorly predictive of volume responsiveness in critically ill patients. Dynamic parameters that vary with the respiratory cycle are better predictors in such patients.

Inferior Vena Cava Size

The widest and the narrowest diameters of the IVC are measured in the M mode (Fig. 5.8). Several criteria are used to assess volume responsiveness based on the change in diameter of the IVC during the respiratory cycle.

Inferior Vena Cava Diameter Variation

$$[(Maximum\ IVC\ diameter - minimum\ IVC\ diameter)/mean\ IVC\ diameter] \times 100$$

An IVC diameter variation of more than 12% is considered to indicate volume responsiveness.

IVC Distensibility Index

$$[(Maximum\ IVC\ diameter - minimum\ IVC\ diameter)/minimum\ IVC\ diameter] \times 100$$

An IVC distensibility index of more than 18% indicates volume responsiveness. Most of the evidence for assessment of volume responsiveness using the IVC diameter is for patients who are on a fully controlled mode with no spontaneous respiratory effort.

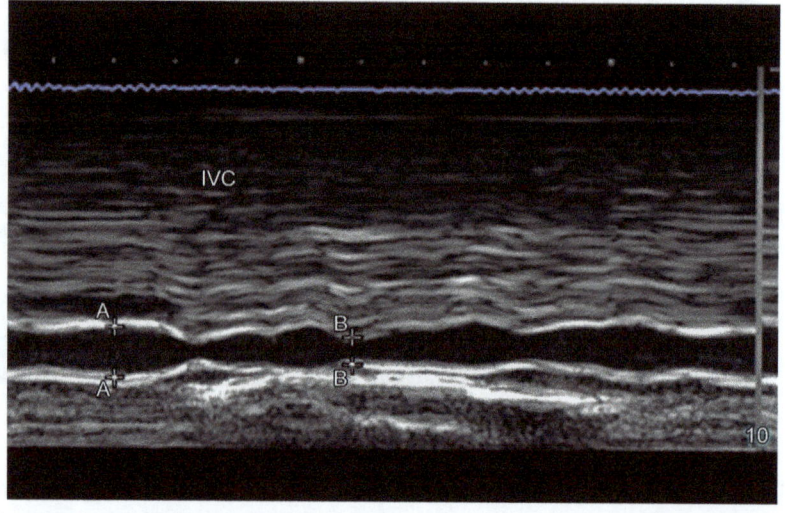

Fig. 5.8: Inferior vena cava (IVC) diameters on M mode: A-A is maximum diameter and B-B is minimum diameter.

Velocity–Time Integral of the Aorta and Stroke Volume

Volume responsiveness can also be assessed using stroke volume variation (SVV). Estimation of stroke volume (SV) is from the A5C view. The sample volume cursor is placed at the LVOT. PW Doppler is applied with the cursor in this position to obtain a velocity trace of the LVOT (Fig. 5.9).

The velocity-time integral (VTI) is measured by tracing out the waveform. The next step is to measure the aortic diameter (d) on the PLAX view. SV is calculated based on the following formula:

$$Stroke\ volume = VTI \times [3.14 \times (d/2)^2]$$

Stroke volume variation is measured using the formula:

$$(Maximum\ SV - minimum\ SV)/mean\ SV \times 100$$

An SVV of more than 12% indicates volume responsiveness.

Lung Ultrasound and Volume Status

There are typical features on ultrasonography that suggests excessive interstitial and intra-alveolar edema. Characteristic "B" lines are seen that radiate from the pleural line, extend to the bottom of the frame, and obliterating "A" lines along the way. More than three "B" lines per field suggest excessive fluid in the lungs (Fig. 5.10); and further fluid loading may not be appropriate in this situation.

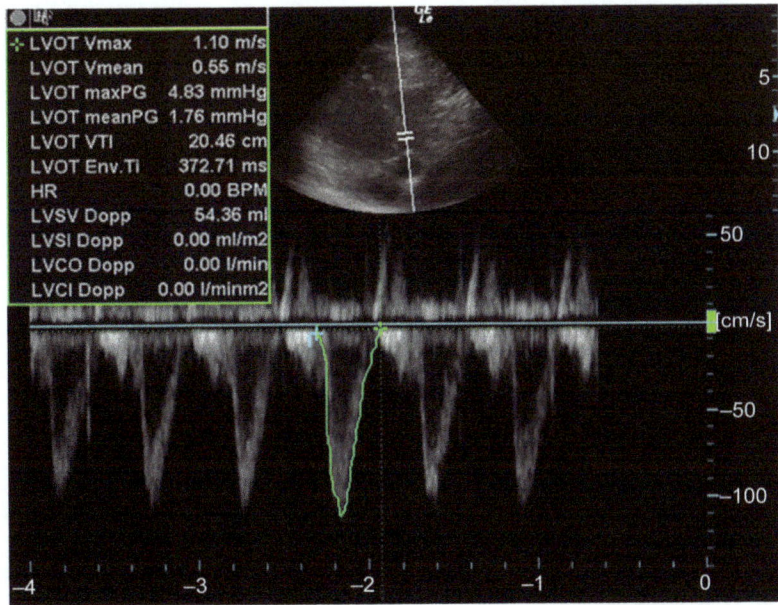

Fig. 5.9: Measurement of the velocity—time integral of the left ventricular outflow tract by pulse wave Doppler.

COMPREHENSIVE ASSESSMENT OF THE HEMODYNAMIC STATUS USING ULTRASONOGRAPHY

An algorithmic approach, as shown in Flowchart 5.1, enables a quick bedside assessment of the hemodynamic status and tailors appropriate therapeutic intervention. This assessment begins with evaluation of cardiac function, presence of pericardial collection, and continues with the assessment of volume responsiveness and signs of fluid overload in the lungs.

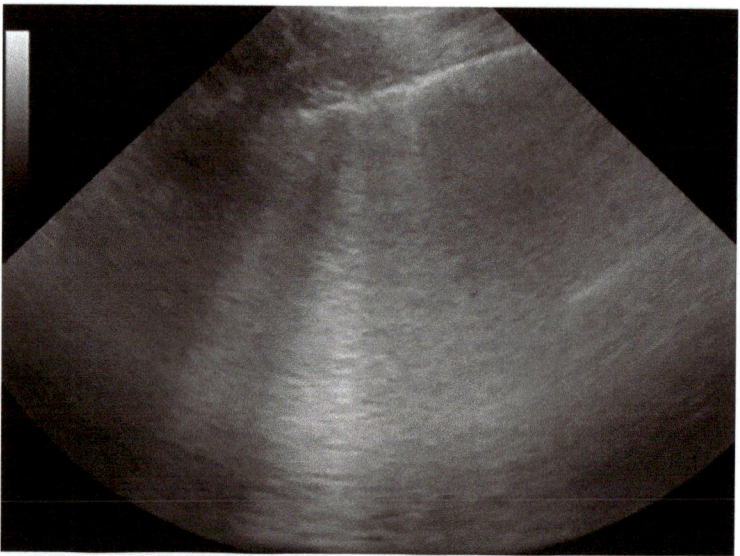

Fig. 5.10: "B" lines suggestive of excessive lung water.

Flowchart 5.1: An algorithmic bedside approach to a hemodynamically unstable patient.

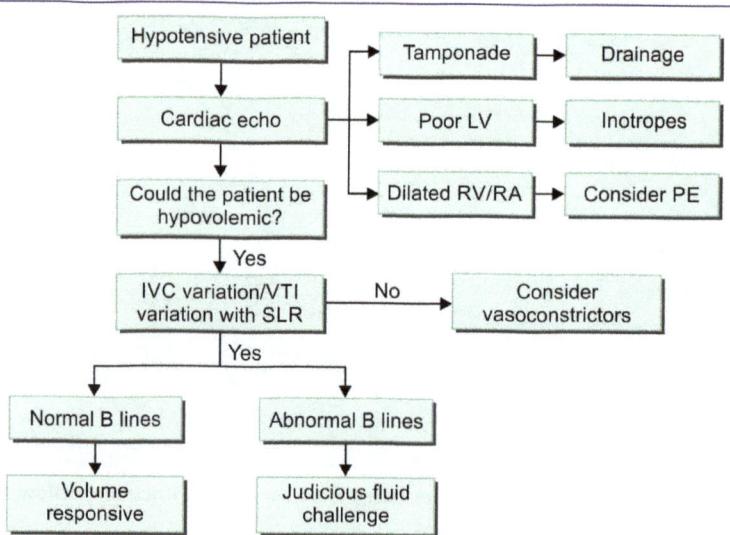

(IVC: inferior vena cava; LV: left ventricular; RA: right atrium; RV: right ventricular; VTI: volume–time integral)

Part 2: Focused Hemodynamic Assessment at Bedside—Interpretations, Fluid Management, and Basic Eyeballing Principles

Jayant Shelgaonkar

INTRODUCTION

Point-of-care ultrasound (POCUS) is emerging as an invaluable and helpful bedside tool to enable accurate decision making in critically ill patients, while the CT scan remains the gold standard for evaluation of many disease processes, considerable risks exist during transport of such patients for the scan. Bedside clinical examination can be complimented by using the ultrasonography for monitoring and diagnosing the condition and therapeutic interventions in a rapidly deteriorating critically ill patient.

With transthoracic echocardiographic examination, we can assess the heart's structures, evaluate functioning, and perform hemodynamically important assessments. An intensive care physician can perform focused echocardiography and obtain relevant hemodynamic parameters following protocolized approach for optimizing care of the patient. Transesophageal studies may be required, if we fail to get good transthoracic windows or for better evaluation of complicated cardiac lesion and artificial valves/devices.

Broad indications for POCUS in the critical care unit:
- Unexplained hypotension/shock in the intensive care unit (ICU)
- Assessing for fluid responsiveness and fluid deficits
- Evaluation for cardiac tamponade
- Evaluation of pulmonary embolism
- Unexplained hypoxemia in the ICU/respiratory insufficiency
- Evaluation of postoperative complications (cardiothoracic and other)
- Right ventricular studies for dysfunction.

BASIC ECHOCARDIOGRAPHIC VIEWS

In the mechanically ventilated patient, it sometimes becomes difficult to obtain the views because of the lung movements. In this scenario, reducing the ventilator pressures (positive-end expiratory and inspiratory briefly may improve visualization of the structures). If for some reason we are unable to get good conventional views, we could attempt to visualize the structures with the subcostal view. To obtain the subcostal view, the probe is placed in the subxiphoid area slightly to the right with the marker point pointing to the left at 3–5 O'clock position.

In some patients, particularly during cardiopulmonary resuscitation, this may be the only available echo window possible without interrupting the chest compressions for significant time.

ASSESSMENT OF VOLUME STATUS

Patients with impending organ failures pose many daunting challenges to the intensivist; main among these challenges is the one regarding fluid administration, as infusion of excess fluids may or may not produce a desired increase in the cardiac output. We assume uniform cardiac contractility during the fluid transfusion; hence, the SV changes to fluid challenges are governed by changes in the ventricular end-diastolic volumes.

Assuming a uniform cardiac contractility, Patterson et al. and Guyton et al. have described the relationship between SV and ventricular end-diastolic volume.

If the ventricular end-diastolic volume is on the lower side, administration of fluids rapidly increases the SV.[1,2] This reflects as an increased cardiac output and oxygen delivery to the tissues. However, once the subject reaches a plateau for the ventricular end-diastolic volume, further preload stress with intravenous fluids will be less likely to increase cardiac output and may even have deleterious effects.[3,4]

It is crucial that the intensivist makes most use of the tools in their grasp to judge the possible requirements of more fluids, which would cause positive hemodynamic effects like better cardiac output, better oxygen delivery, and organ failure reversal; or negative effects like tissue edema, more mortality, or worsening hypoxia.[5]

Bedside assessments, which change preloads rapidly, are now being recognized as more judgmental than static measures.[2] Commonly used measures presently are the passive leg raising (PLR) test and respiratory variation in thoracic pressure.

If a patient who is not on medications for low-blood pressure, post-bilateral PLR for 1 minute has an increase in preload; and consequent raise in blood pressure through recruitment of blood pooled in the legs, he is considered a "responder", i.e. the patient may show suitable response to fluid boluses. This technique is therefore best suited to patients who are not yet on vasopressors with normal intrathoracic pressures and those without significant abdominal pathology (as increased intra-abdominal pressures interfere with the analysis).

In mechanically ventilated patients with no respiratory effort, pulse pressure fluctuations are seen as a surrogate marker of the fluid depleted state; the more the variations the better chances the patient may have of responding to fluids and, hence, increase the cardiac output. This method is fallacious when there is an irregular heart rate as in arrhythmias and severe tachycardias.

Changes in the intrathoracic pressures with respiration cause changes in the diameters of both superior vena cava (SVC) and IVC. These changes depend on the level of pressure change within the thorax and also on the compliance of the vena cava. Usually, a positive pressure will increase and negative pressure will reduce the diameter of the vena cava. Hence, a large distended vena cava means the patient is less likely to be fluid responsive and the opposite is true for a completely collapsing vena cava.

The measurements are done around 1–2 cm from the right atrial junction, usually distal to the hepatic veins.[6-11]

ASSESSING VOLUME RESPONSE AT THE PATIENTS BEDSIDE

Monitoring SVV by doing the PLR with Point-of-care Ultrasound

The PLR is one of the easiest and reliable methods available, which can be done both by the patients side (patient breathes spontaneously) and also if the patient is mechanically ventilated.

A recent meta-analysis showed a strong global predictive value of the PLR and a reasonably good sensitivity and specificity.

The preload dependency is tested in this maneuver. Initially, the patient is positioned in a semirecumbent position with the head of the bed 30–45° above the horizontal. The PLR maneuver consists of swiftly moving the lower end of the bed to raise the lower extremities to 30–45° above the horizontal while lowering the head of the bed to 0° (supine). This process transfers blood rapidly from the legs and the splanchnic reservoir of circulation to the intrathoracic compartment, rapidly causing an increase in the preload, and thereby testing the preload dependency of the heart.[12,13]

By this maneuver, around 250–350 mL of blood is mobilized from the lower extremities to the heart and also is entirely reversible. It is absolutely imperative that this maneuver must be done from the semirecumbent position because this will increase the blood shift and accentuates the changes in cardiac output as compared with a subject who starts in the supine position. These changes in the cardiac output can be detected a few minutes after the maneuver using bedside echocardiography.

Irregular heart rhythms should not usually affect the diagnostic performance of the test because the effects of the maneuver are measured over multiple heartbeats and also multiple respiratory cycles, hence, possible negating and distorting effects of the same.[14] However, large studies are required in this field.

Patients with significant intra-abdominal hypertension may cause inaccuracies in the test.[15]

Using Ultrasound to Monitor Stroke Volume while receiving Controlled Mechanical Ventilation

A patient on the ventilator has many complicated situations, hence, aortic flow variations may be a better measure of the clinical status, as SVV is a parameter, which correlates with fluid responsiveness. A variation during the respiratory cycle greater than 12% is accurately predictive of the fluid. An A5C view using pulsed Doppler imaging is used to get the required measurements. Patients with irregular heart rates and right ventricular dysfunction are limiting factors to the test.[16]

Measurements of aortic blood flow during mechanical ventilation are of limited utility in patients subject to "open lung" ventilator strategies, which reduce the pressure changes within the pleural cavity.

IVC Size and Its Variability

Controlled Ventilation

Studying the IVC, looking for the variability, and measuring the diameters are best done on M-mode images of a longitudinal view of the IVC, which can be obtained from the subcostal view. Several studies have analyzed the IVC in ICU patients on controlled mechanical ventilation.[17-20] All of them have conclude the restricted utility of the static measures of the IVC diameter in predicting fluid responsiveness. In contrast, the change in IVC diameter induced by intrathoracic pressure swings during mechanical ventilation is useful. Using the ratio between maximal size minus minimum size to the average of these two values, (Collapsibility Index) a variation more than 12% was associated with an increase of cardiac output after fluid infusion.[19]

An 18% was the cutoff value by using the ratio of the maximal size minus the minimum size divided by the minimum size (distensibility index).[17] Shortcomings to these approaches can be caused by raised intra-abdominal pressures, tidal volumes, and patients inspiration efforts, while spontaneous breaths are taken.[21]

Spontaneously Breathing Patient

Some recent articles have shown a good correlation of change in IVC diameter with respiratory effort in healthy people. Hence, a patient on spontaneous breathing mode of ventilator can have variable figures based on the level of positive pressure applied.[22] The above fact has to be taken into account while treating and interpreting awake patients who are to be transfused with fluids.[23]

The variations in the IVC diameter with respirations may create many false-positive and false-negative situations, mainly due to patient ventilator settings and changes, hyperinflation of the lungs, reduced venous return by certain cardiac conditions, and raised intra-abdominal pressures.[24]

Assessment of Left Ventricular End-diastolic Area

If in the PLAX view and sometimes PSAX at papillary muscle level view if you see complete obliteration of the LV cavity in systole at the level of the papillary muscle, many call this the "kissing sign" or kissing ventricle sign, which is highly suggestive of the hypovolemic state. Performing a more objective assessment can be done by measurement of the LV end-diastolic area by tracing the endocardial border. This, however, may be cumbersome to carry out due to poor echo windows and can also consume valuable time. Some studies propose the left ventricular end-diastolic area (LVEDA) as a good predictor of volume responsiveness,[25] but very few studies support this finding.[26,27] Variability of the LVEDA occurs between patients depending on the patients cardiac condition and physiology and, hence, absolute values are difficult to find.

ASSESSMENT OF LV FUNCTION

LV Ejection Fraction

Ejection fraction (EF) is the percentage of blood ejected from the ventricle during systole in relation to the total end-diastolic volume in the left ventricle. We can visually judge LV function on the basis of how much change in the size occurs during systole.

When the cardiac function is affected, less blood will be ejected and the EF will reduce. EF is also dependent on the size of the ventricle. So, if the ventricle size is small (as in hypovolemia), compensation occurs by increasing the contractility. The EF will be more than normal (hypercontractile heart).

Conventional echographic methods do not assess the functional capacity or contractile reserve of the ventricle, hence, only reliability on EF is discouraged.

Various methods have been proposed to assess the LV function and these include evaluation by fractional shortening, the Simpson method, and just eyeballing.

Fractional Shortening

This is usually calculated from M-mode imaging, and linear measurements taken shortcomings to this method are seen with regional wall motion abnormalities. Asymmetric sizes of the ventricles LV volume may be a better marker of LV size than linear dimension measured at the LV base.

To calculate the fractional shortening the M-mode marker is placed in the LV just beyond the MV leaflets. A trace with LV chamber diameters in both systole and diastole is obtained. Based on the end-systolic and end-diastolic diameters, we calculate the fractional shortening. This shortening fraction reflects the left ventricle systolic function (only if the left ventricle shape is normal and there is no wall motion abnormality) (Tables 5.1 and 5.2).

Ejection Fraction

This is calculated as the difference between end-diastolic and end-systolic LV volume, divided by the end-diastolic LV volume. A commonly used method for volume measurements is the biplane method of disks (modified Simpson's rule). The LV volume (total) is calculated by totaling the sum of all the "stack of elliptical disks", which comprise the left ventricle.

Measurement of the LV volumes is made from the A4C/apical 2-chamber (A2C) views by tracing endocardial borders of the LV. The echocardiography machine by an inbuilt calculation will give the volume of the cavity.

Table 5.1: Fractional shortening.

Parameter	Formula	Abbreviation	Values (range)
LV internal dimension in diastole (cm)	—	LVIDd	3.6–5.6
LV internal dimension in systole (cm)	—	LVIDs	2.3–3.9
Fractional shortening (%)	(LVIDd – LVIDs)/LVIDd	FS	27–42

(FS: fractional shortening; LVIDd: left ventricular internal diameter end diastole; LVIDs: left ventricular internal diameter end systole)

Table 5.2: Correlation of fractional shortening and LV dysfunction.

Shortening fraction	%
Normal	25–45
Mild	20–25
Moderate	15–20
Severe	<15

Table 5.3: Normal values.

	Hyperdynamic LV function	Normal LV function	Mild LV dysfunction	Moderate LV dysfunction	Severe LV dysfunction
EF (%)	<65	55–65	45–55	30–45	30>

(EF: ejection fraction; LV: left ventricle)

Table 5.4: Grading of left ventricular function.

Hyperdynamic	>70%
Normal	69–55%
Borderline	54–50%
Mildly reduced	50–40%
Moderately reduced	40–30%
Severely reduced	<30%

Barring wall motion abnormalities, the EF can be estimated from either A4C or A2C, both views to be done, if regional wall motion abnormalities exist (Table 5.3).[28,29]

Pitfalls:
- An accurate A4C view, which is not foreshortened and in which both mitral and tricuspid leaflets with full atria are seen.
- Accurate tracing of the endocardial border with good image quality is required.
- Both systolic and diastolic volumes have to be measured from the same cardiac cycle, and if the heart rate is irregular, an average of measurements over several cycles is taken.[29]

Eyeballing of Left Ventricle

Even with limited training, a reasonably accurate estimation of the LV function is possible and this has also been proven to be quite.[29] It is possible to assess the LV function from all echocardiographic windows for better and more accurate results, at least two different views are recommended in case of a doubt.

Structures observed during the eyeballing exercise include the endocardial movements, mitral annular motion in longitudinal plane, shape of the ventricle, and myocardial thickening.

The following scheme may be used to grade LV function (Table 5.4).

MEASUREMENT OF CARDIAC OUTPUT

Stroke volume is calculated based on a simple formula, which is related to the flow of fluids through a cylinder. The volume of fluid flowing through the cylinder in unit time is given by the multiplication of the mean flow velocity V and the area of cross-section of the cylinder. This principle is now applied to the heart and we regard the aorta as a cylinder whose area we can measure. Since blood flow through this conduit is pulsatile and varies with time during the full LV ejection, all individual velocities have to be assimilated as the VTI.

Measurement of the area under the curve will tell us the distance blood has moved travelling at these velocities for a specified amount of time. Next, we calculate the volume of the cylinder by multiplying the area of the LVOT and the length the blood travels and you get the SV (i.e. amount of blood ejected per beat). The SV multiplied by the heart rate gives us the cardiac output (expressed as L/min). The cardiac index is calculated by dividing the cardiac output by the body surface area.

Procedure

Step 1

On PLAX view, measure the LVOT diameter.

Step 2

Visualize the LVOT by either A5C or apical 3-chamber view (A3C) views and use PW Doppler to obtain a satisfactory waveform. The PW gate width should be 2–4 mm.

Step 3

The PW waveform tracing is then taken.

A trace is made along the edges of the velocity to measure the area under the curve (the VTI expressed in cm) (Fig. 5.11).

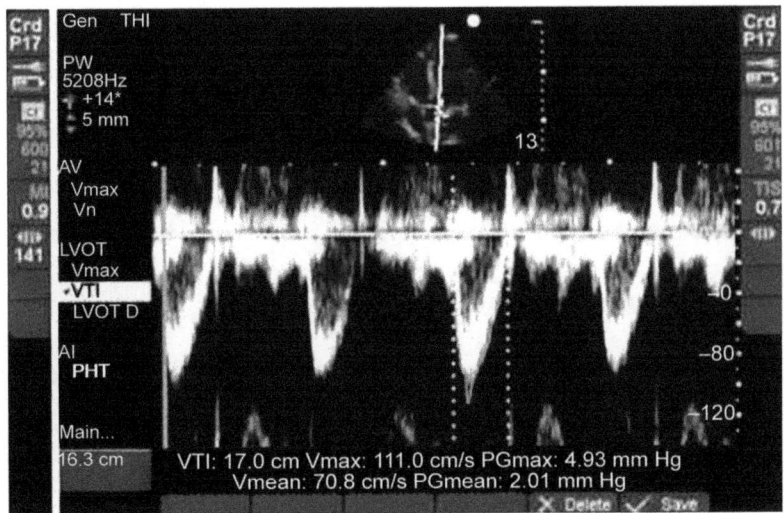

Fig. 5.11: Measurement of velocity-time integral (VTI).

$$LVOT\ area = \pi \times r^2\ or\ \pi \times (d/2)^2$$
$$Stroke\ volume = \pi \times (d^2/4) \times VTI$$
$$Cardiac\ output = Stroke\ volume \times Heart\ rate$$

The VTI variability with respiration could be indicative of volume responsiveness and this has been validated in patients undergoing coronary artery surgery, under closed chest conditions.[28]

ASSESSMENT OF RIGHT VENTRICULAR FUNCTION

The right ventricle is the most anterior cardiac chamber of the heart. It consists of the inlet, trabeculated apical myocardium, and infundibulum or conus.

The inlet is made up of tricuspid valve, chordae tendineae, and papillary muscles.

The shape of the right ventricle is like a triangle when side view is done and like a crescent or sail when seen in cross-section.

Size of the RV can be assessed by A4C view and measurements of the area from this view. The ratio of the RV:LV area is used to grade RV dilatation.

The normal ratio is less than 0.6; dilatation is considered moderate—if it is 0.6–1.0 and severe—if more than 1.0.[30] This can also be done by eyeballing. In cases of RV overload as in acute respiratory distress syndrome (ARDS), pulmonary embolism, and high ventilator pressures, the septum shifts to the left and the left ventricle assumes a "D" shape. This has been described by some as the "D" sign.[31,32]

TRICUSPID ANNULAR PLANE SYSTOLIC EXCURSION OR TRICUSPID ANNULAR MOTION

The systolic movement of the base of the RV-free wall provides one of the most visibly obvious movements on normal echocardiography. Tricuspid annular plane systolic excursion (TAPSE) or tricuspid annular motion (TAM) is a method to measure the distance of systolic excursion of the RV annular segment along its longitudinal plane, from a standard A4C window. It represents longitudinal function of the right ventricle. This image is acquired by placing M mode through the tricuspid annulus and measuring the amount of longitudinal motion of the annulus at peak systole.

Normal values are displacement of annulus of more than 1.75 cm.

Displacement between 1.5 cm and 1.75 cm represents borderline right ventricular dysfunction.

Less than 1.5 cm represents RV dysfunction.

TRICUSPID ANNULUS PEAK SYSTOLIC VELOCITY OR DOPPLER TISSUE IMAGING RIGHT VENTRICLE TRICUSPID ANNULUS PEAK SYSTOLIC VELOCITY

To perform this measure, an A4C window is used with a tissue Doppler (TDI) mode region of interest highlighting the RV-free wall. The pulsed Doppler sample volume is placed in either

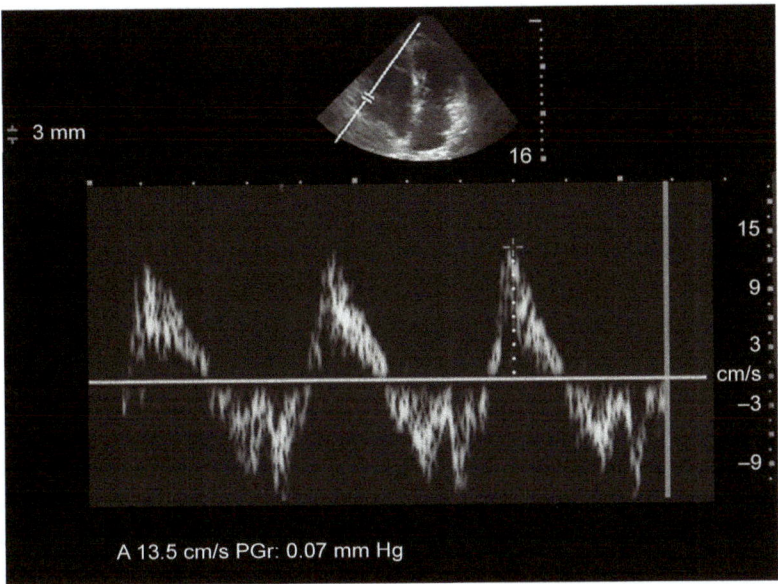

Fig. 5.12: Measurement of tricuspid annulus peak systolic velocity (TAPSV).

the tricuspid annulus or the middle of the basal segment of the RV-free wall. Velocity less than 10 cm per second should raise the suspicion of abnormal RV function.[33] This correlates with right ventricular ejection fraction (RVEF) less than 50% measured by Simpson's rule method with a sensitivity of 60% and a specificity of 90% (Fig. 5.12).

Echocardiographic assessment of the right ventricle has been largely qualitative, primarily because of the difficulty with assessing RV volumes because of its unusual shape. Hence, there are minimal quantitative data overall on RV size and function in normal controls and in disease states.

Part 3: Critical Care Ultrasound—Valvular Assessment, Regional Wall Assessment, and Diastolic Dysfunction Assessment

Charudutt Vaity, Rahul Pandit

FOCUSED ASSESSMENT OF CARDIAC VALVES

Echocardiography is an important tool to assess valvular abnormalities. Color flow and PW Doppler assessment can provide valuable information to assist clinical management.[34-36]

Doppler Evaluation of the Valves

The apical view is best view for quick Doppler examination of the valves. The Doppler beam is parallel as possible to the direction of blood flow through mitral, tricuspid, and AVs. Lets

revise the different Doppler modes, which can be used. Doppler echo uses Doppler principle to derive velocity information. The three commonly used Doppler echo techniques are:
1. *Continuous wave Doppler*: There are two piezoelectric crystals—one transmitting continuously and the other receiving continuously. This allows for measuring high velocities but this limits the ability to precisely localize the flow signal (Figs. 5.13A and B). Continuous wave Doppler is used to assess for stenosis of cardiac valves.
2. *Pulse wave Doppler*: Single crystal is used, which alternates in first to transmit the signal and then to receive it. This helps in to localize a flow disturbance or to measure blood velocity from a small region. However, while localizing the region, there is limit on the highest velocities, which can be measured. This limit is called as Nyquist limit. Nyquist limit is half of the pulse repetition frequency (pulse is the signal from the crystal). PW Doppler is mainly used for assessment of diastolic function (Figs. 5.14A and B).
3. *Color flow mapping*: This is modified version of two-dimensional (2D) echo with PW Doppler. The blood velocity and direction are calculated at multiple points, which is the then represented in a color coded. The velocities away from the transducer are color coded in blue and toward the transducer are coded in red. This is known as BART convention (Blue Away Red Toward). Progressive lighter shades are used to show higher velocities. Color reversal occurs above threshold velocity by the phenomenon of aliasing (Fig. 5.15). Color flow Doppler is useful in assessment of regurgitation and shunts.

Vena Contracta

It is important to understand the concept of vena contracta to be able to quantify regurgitant lesions. When assessing the regurgitant valve by color flow mapping, the narrowest region of

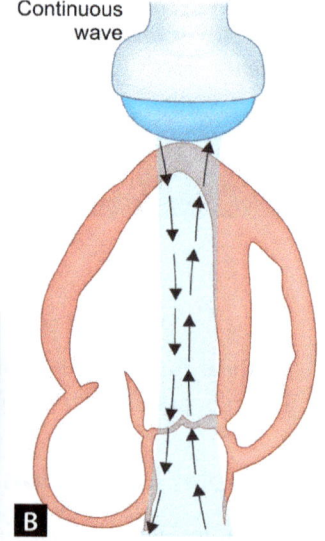

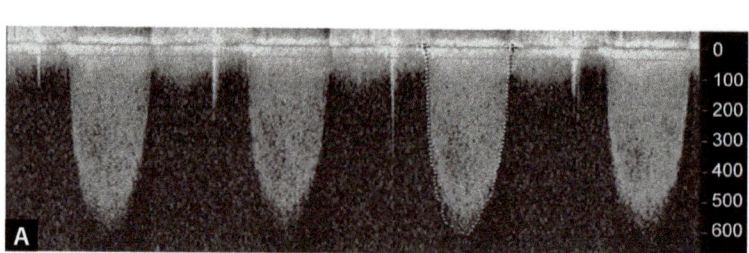

Figs. 5.13A and B: Continuous wave Doppler.

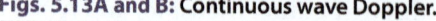

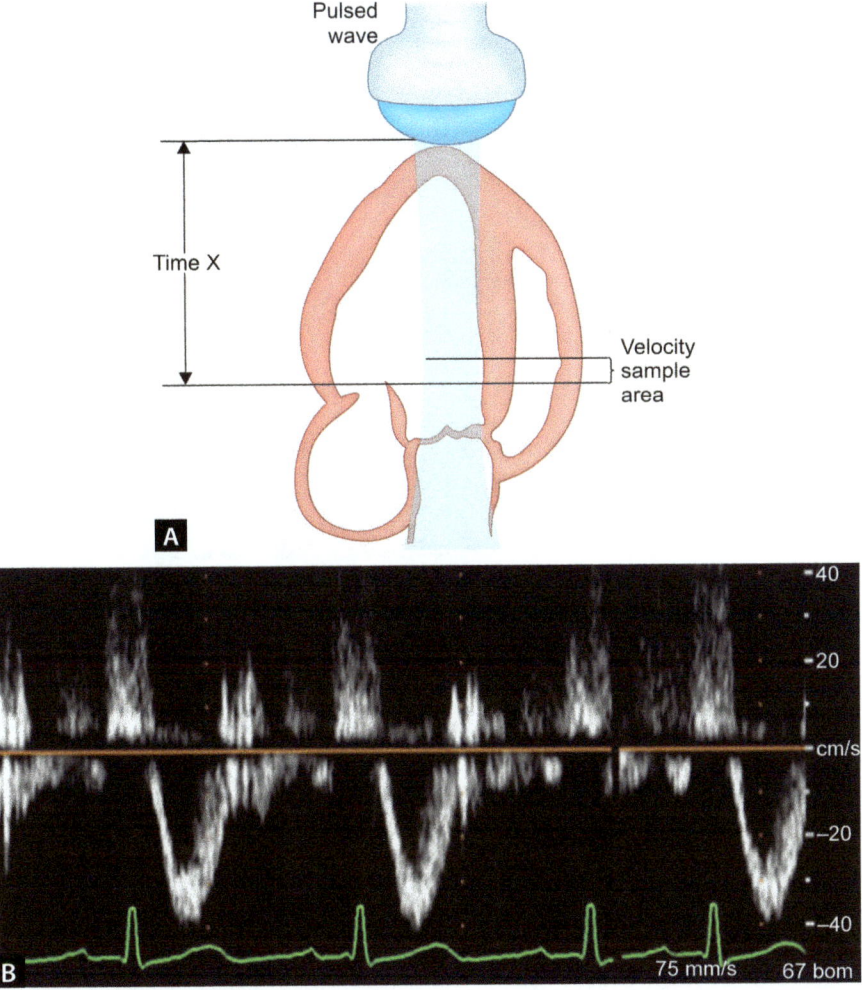

Figs. 5.14A and B: Pulse wave Doppler.

the jet just below the orifice of the regurgitant valve is called as vena contracta (Fig. 5.16). Vena contracta measurements are useful in assessment of severity of mitral, tricuspid, and aortic regurgitation.

Approach to Echo Assessment of Valvular Lesion

- *Step 1*: 2D echo to look for structural abnormalities like valve movement, vegetations, calcifications, etc.
- *Step 2*: Apply color Doppler over the area of concern to assess for regurgitation.
- *Step 3*: Uses continuous wave Doppler to assess for stenosis gradient.
- *Step 4*: If possible, measure vena contracta.

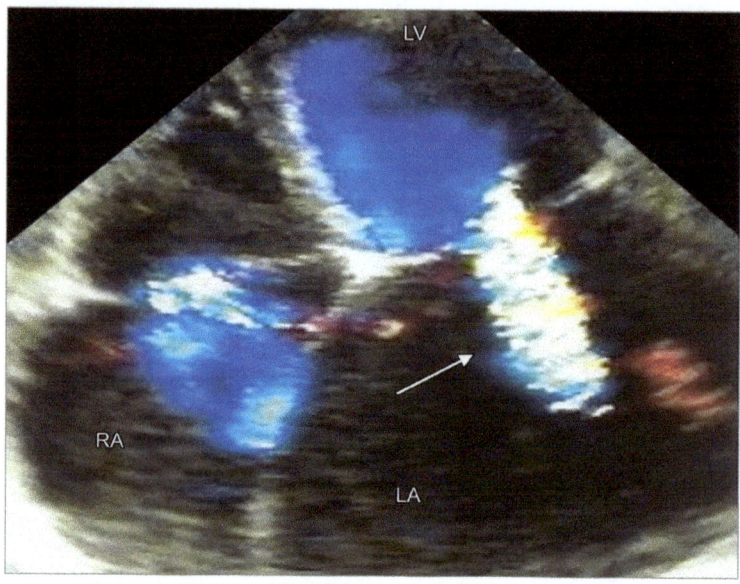

Fig. 5.15: Color flow mapping.
(LA: left atrium; LV: left ventricular; RA: right atrium)

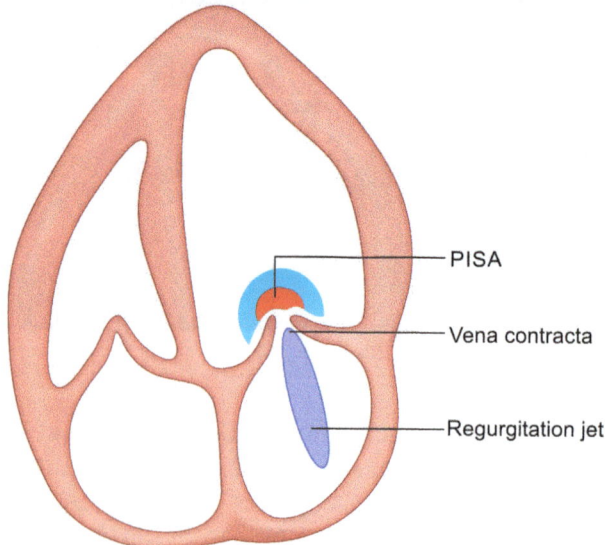

Fig. 5.16: Vena contracta.
(PISA: proximal isovelocity surface area)

Mitral Stenosis

On 2D echo, the MV leaflets can be seen to be thickened. Fusion of the anterior and posterior leaflet may give characteristic "bent-knee appearance" (Fig. 5.17).

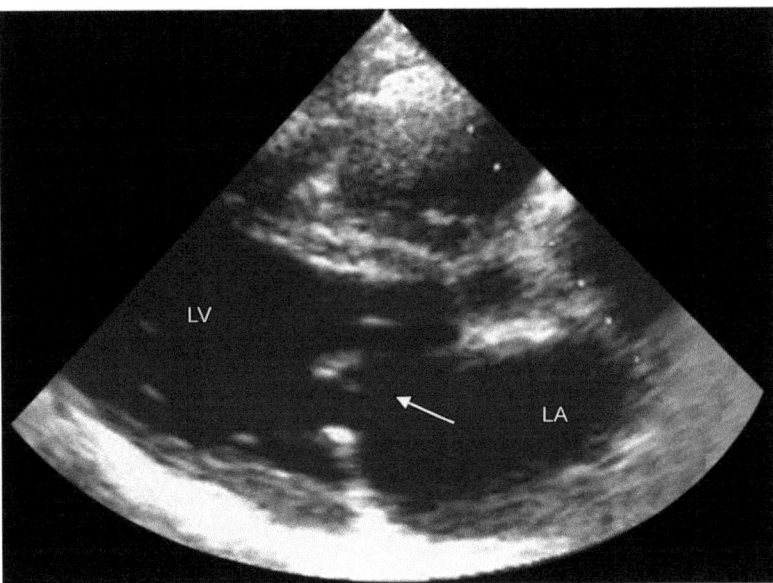

Fig. 5.17: Bent-knee appearance of mitral stenosis.

On PSAX view, the MV leaflets can be seen to open and close in "fish mouth pattern".

By applying the continuous wave Doppler, it is possible to assess the severity of stenosis. In normal valve, the blood flow velocity will peak rapidly and also fall away quickly as the pressures between LA and LV equalize. In stenosed valve, the pressure gradient has to maintain for longer period of time to push blood through narrow orifice (Fig. 5.18). Therefore, there is inverse relationship between mitral valve area (MVA) and the time taken for the pressure gradient to fall away to half its peak value (pressure half time-T).

$$MVA = 220/T \text{ (220 is the constant)}$$

Mitral Regurgitation

On 2D echo, apart from seeing abnormalities in the MV like MV prolapse, vegetations, and there can also be features of chronic mitral regurgitation (MR) in LV, which become dilated, volume overloaded, and hyperdynamic. The LA also becomes dilated.

By applying color Doppler, one can look for the extent of the MR jet. Vena contracta can be measured as mentioned before. There is good correlation between the width of the vena contracta and severity of MR. Continuous wave Doppler will show dense signal. The intensity of jet greater with more severe MR (Fig. 5.19).

Aortic Stenosis

Using 2D echo parasternal long axis and short axis and A5C views, we can get information on AV structural abnormalities like bicuspid AV, calcifications, thickening, etc. Apart from this, we

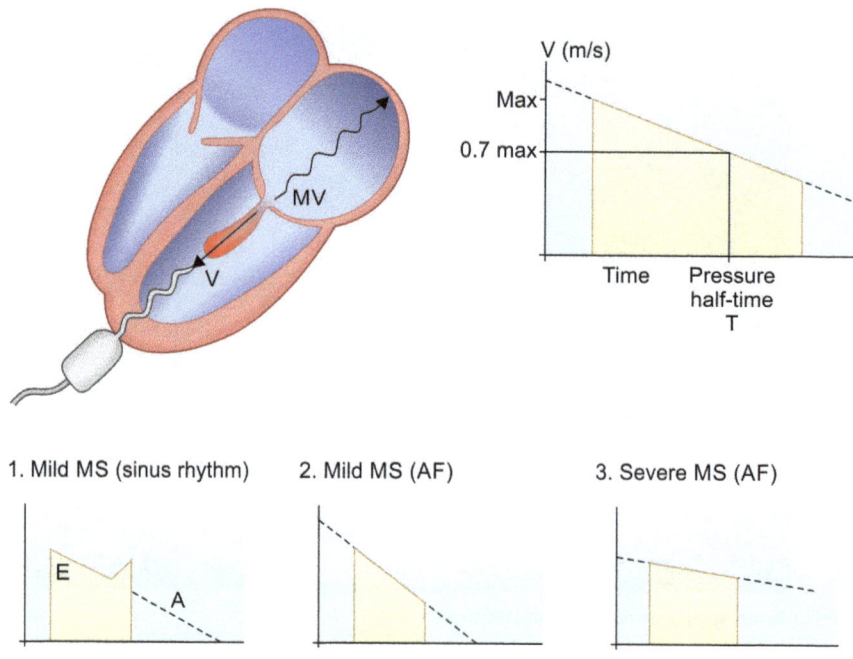

Fig. 5.18: Mitral stenosis (MS)—Doppler assessment.

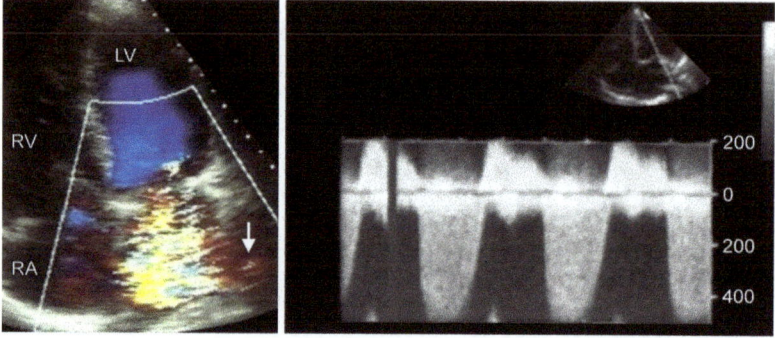

Fig. 5.19: Severe mitral regurgitation.

can also see features of chronic AS like left ventricular hypertrophy; LV can get dilated, if heart failure has occurred and is a poor prognostic indicator. There can be poststenotic dilatation of the aorta.

Continuous wave Doppler is very useful in assessing the severity of AS by estimating the pressure gradient (Fig. 5.20). The severity of aortic stenosis (AS) correlates with the valve area, peak velocity, peak pressure gradient, and mean pressure gradient. One has to be aware of the relationship of AV pressure gradient and cardiac output. They can be overestimated in high-output states and underestimated in low-output states.

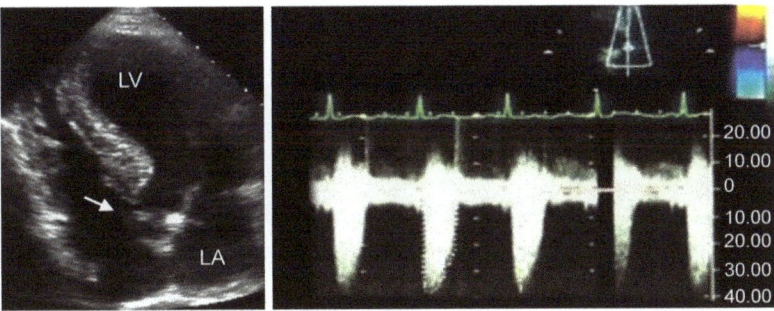

Fig. 5.20: Doppler in aortic stenosis/aortic regurgitation.

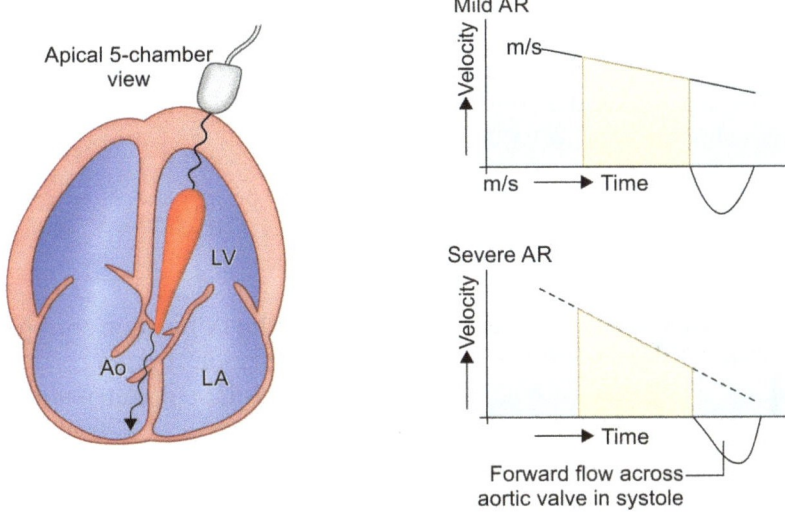

Fig. 5.21: Doppler assessment of aortic regurgitation.
(Ao: aorta; LA: left atrium; LV: left ventricular)

Aortic Regurgitation

Two-dimensional echo is not directly useful to diagnose AR but may indicate underlying etiology like dilated aortic root, bicuspid valve, vegetation, etc. and also aid in assessment of effects of AR like LV dilatation.

Doppler is very useful in detecting AR and assessing its severity. Color flow Doppler will identify the jet of AR entering the LV. This can be seen best in PSAX and A5C. Vena contracta can be measured and shows good correlation with severity. Measuring the vena contracta can be limited when there are multiple AR jets. Jet width and length also indicate severity.

Continuous wave Doppler is also helpful in quantifying the severity of AR. The slope and intensity of the continuous Doppler signal can indicate severity (Fig. 5.21). The greater the slope, the more severe the AR. This can also be expressed as pressure half-time.

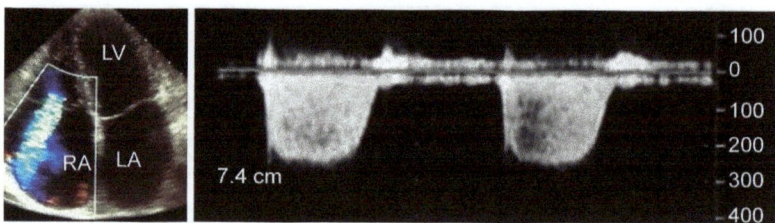

Fig. 5.22: Tricuspid regurgitation—color flow and continuous wave Doppler.
(LA: left atrium; LV: left ventricular; RA: right atrium)

Pulmonary Artery Systolic Pressure from Tricuspid Regurgitation

Pulmonary artery systolic pressure (PASP) is equal to right ventricular systolic pressure (RVSP). RVSP can be easily estimated from measuring the maximum velocity of the TR jet (TR_{vmax}) by using color flow Doppler and continuous wave Doppler (Fig. 5.22). The value of PASP can be calculated by using the formula PASP = $4 (TR_{vmax})_2$ + RAP.

FOCUSED CARDIAC ULTRASOUND: REGIONAL WALL BASICS

Introduction

Most common referral to echocardiography is to assess the LV function and specifically assess regional wall motion abnormality (RWMA). The information is often correlated with other clinical findings and electrocardiograph (ECG). It is important to understand the myocardial mechanics before assessing LV function and regional wall motion. The left ventricle not only contracts in radial direction, but also has a shortening of its length and a circumferential motion as well. The inward motion of endocardium and thickening of myocardium during LV systole is most often used to determine the wall motion.

Eyeballing

The most common way of assessment is eyeballing. It has been shown in numerous studies that an experienced echocardiographer will reasonably assess the LV function with eyeballing and give a reasonable estimate of its wall motion and EF.

Following helps in assessment during eyeballing.
- Inward motion of the endocardium
- Thickening of the myocardium
- Longitudinal motion of the mitral annulus
- Geometry of the ventricle.

Regional wall motion abnormality means motion of a particular region of the heart is found to be abnormal on echocardiography. Different types of regional wall motion abnormalities are:
- *Hypokinesia*: Reduced contraction of a region of the heart muscle
- *Akinesia*: A region of the heart muscle is not contracting at all.

- *Hyperkinesia*: A region of the heart muscle is contracting more vigorously than normal.
- *Dyskinesia*: A region of the heart muscle bulges out when the rest of the heart is contracting.

The different regions of the heart are divided as per the arterial territories (Fig. 5.23). PSAX gives a quick guide on RWMA for all three territories.

LV Function Assessment

Usually the assessment is done and reported as hyperdynamic, good LV function, moderate LV dysfunction, or poor or severe LV dysfunction. Most echocardiographs are able to assess and give a number on basis of eyeballing as well. However, a more objective way is to assess the LV systolic function with various techniques available like fractional shortening, Simpson's method, three-dimensional echocardiography, and dP/dt method. The most common used is Simpson's method.

Simpson's Method

It is by far the most commonly used method to determine EF. It can be applied in monoplane and biplane method. The biplane method been the more accurate one, determines the LV

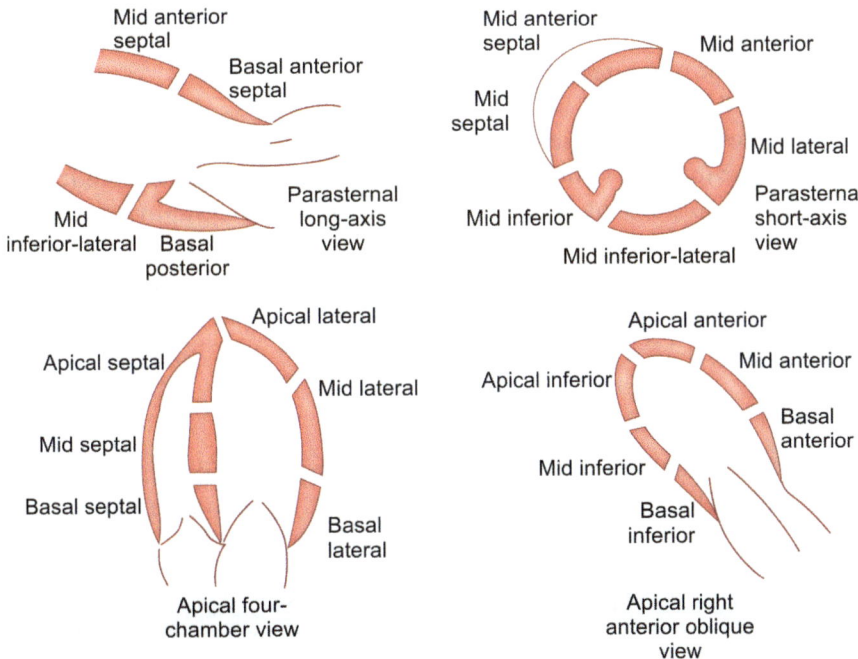

Fig. 5.23: 17-segment model of left ventricular myocardium. Arterial territories are shown.
Source: Adapted from Kondo H, Masuyama T, Ishihara K, et al. Digital subtraction high-frame-rate echocardiography in detecting delayed onset of regional left ventricular relaxation in ischemic heart disease. Circulation. 1995;91:304-12.

volume in A4C view and A2C view. The limiting factor for Simpson's method is image quality; in clinical practice, one would come across numerous situations where image quality may not be adequate to apply Simpson's method.

The formula used is:

$$\text{Ejection fraction} = \frac{\text{End-diastolic volume} - \text{End-systolic volume}}{\text{End-diastolic volume}} \times 100$$

Based on this method, following values, given in Table 5.5, of EF may be reported.

Diastolic Function and Assessment

Diastolic function is often described as filling of the heart during diastole. Since the LV diastole is an active process consisting of four phases:
1. Isovolumetric relaxation
2. Rapid filling phase
3. Diastasis
4. Atrial contraction.

Diastolic function is dependent on both speed of relaxation and compliance of the left ventricle. The four factors, which determine diastolic dysfunction, are as follows:
1. Slow force (or pressure) decay and cellular relengthening rates
2. Increase early filling rates and deceleration
3. Elevated diastolic pressures
4. Poor viscoelasticity of LV fibers.

Several techniques and parameters have been introduced to assess diastolic function of the heart. The complexity of this phenomenon and the difficulties in interpreting these findings have led to confusion among those performing echocardiography as well as those who interpret its results.

The MV inflow seems to be the most commonly used technique and also the physiologically most suitable. However, arrhythmias and other valvular lesions may interfere into the assessment.

Mitral Valve Inflow

The mitral inflow signal visualizes the individual phases of filling as well as displays the contribution of each individual phase in filling. As mitral inflow reflects the pressure difference

Table 5.5: Different values of ejection fraction.

Normal	>55 %
Mild	45–54%
Moderate	30–44%
Severe	<30%

between the atria and the ventricle, any abnormality of diastolic pressure (as in the presence of diastolic dysfunction) in the chambers will affect the velocity and shape of the Doppler inflow signal. Specifically, diastolic dysfunction alters the relationship between early and late filling (E- and A-wave), how rapidly flow velocity declines in early diastole (E-wave deceleration time = DT), and how long it takes for filling of the ventricle to start after the ventricle relaxes (length of the isovolumetric relaxation time = IVRT) (Fig. 5.24).

Normal Diastolic Function

In preserved diastolic function, blood flows and fills the LV in early filling phase thus the E wave is taller than the A wave, the deceleration time is around 140–200 milliseconds and isovolumetric relaxation time is 70–100 mm/s. E/A ratio is between 0.8 and 2.0.

Grade-I Diastolic Dysfunction

A stiff ventricle will impair early filling of the ventricle. Thus, the magnitude of the E wave will decrease. It will take longer for atrial pressure to be high enough to initiate filling. The IVRT will increase (>100 ms) and the DT will also be prolonged (≥240 ms). As less volume is transported into the left ventricle during early filling, more blood is present at the time of atrial contraction. Therefore, atrial contraction will eject more blood into the left ventricle. The A wave will be larger than normal and will typically also be larger than the E wave (E/A ratio ≤ 0.8) (Fig. 5.25).

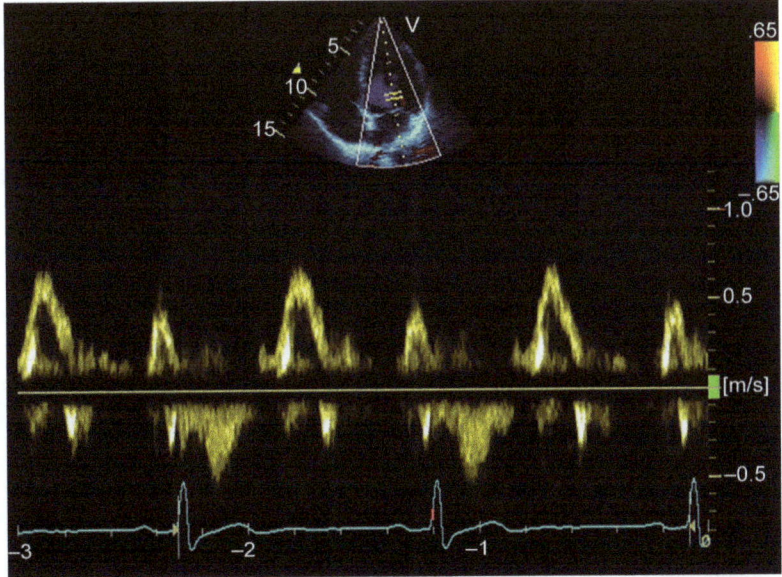

Fig. 5.24: Normal mitral valve inflow showing E and A waves.

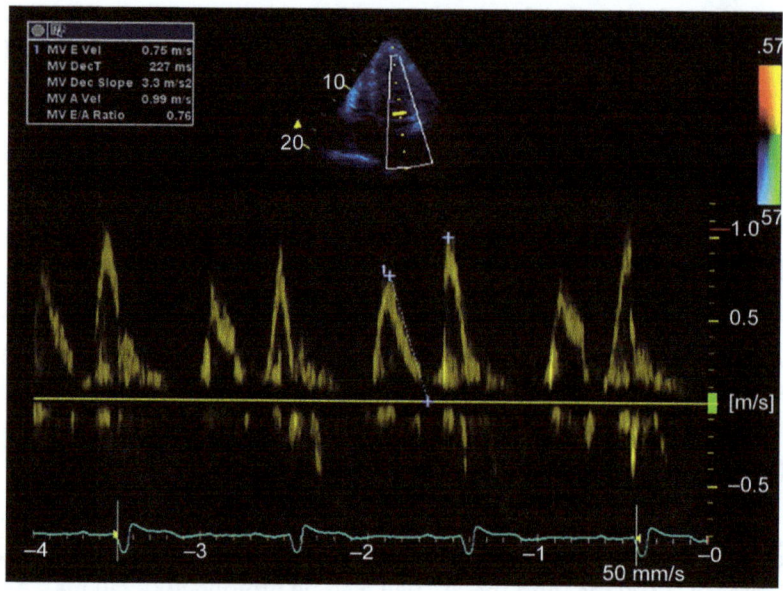

Fig. 5.25: E and A reversal—stage-I dysfunction.

Grade-II Diastolic Dysfunction—Pseudonormal

Progressive diastolic dysfunction causes left atrial pressure to rise. The latter increases the pressure gradient between the LA and the LV and will act as a driving force to fill the ventricle during early diastole. Thus the size of the E wave relative to the A wave will increase, and the E/A ratio will return to the range of 0.8–1.5. DT and IVRT (<90 ms) will also decrease. The spectrum will look very similar to that of "normal" diastolic function. This condition is therefore referred to as "pseudonormal". Pseudonormal filling is classified as grade-II diastolic dysfunction.

Several approaches may be used to distinguish between "normal" and pseudonormal filling: the most common been Valsalva maneuver. It unmasks the pseudonormal trace and reverts back to impaired relaxation—grade-I dysfunction trace.

The other approach is to use TDI imaging at the MV annulus and get the e' and a'. The ratio of E/e' more than 15 will help to unmask pseudonormal dysfunction. Also the mitral annulus TDI will show a trace like stag-I dysfunction mirror image (Figs. 5.26A and B).

Stage-III Diastolic Dysfunction

A further increase in filling pressure will increase the gradient between the LA and the LV during early diastole. The E wave will become even taller and the A wave shorter. The E/A ratio

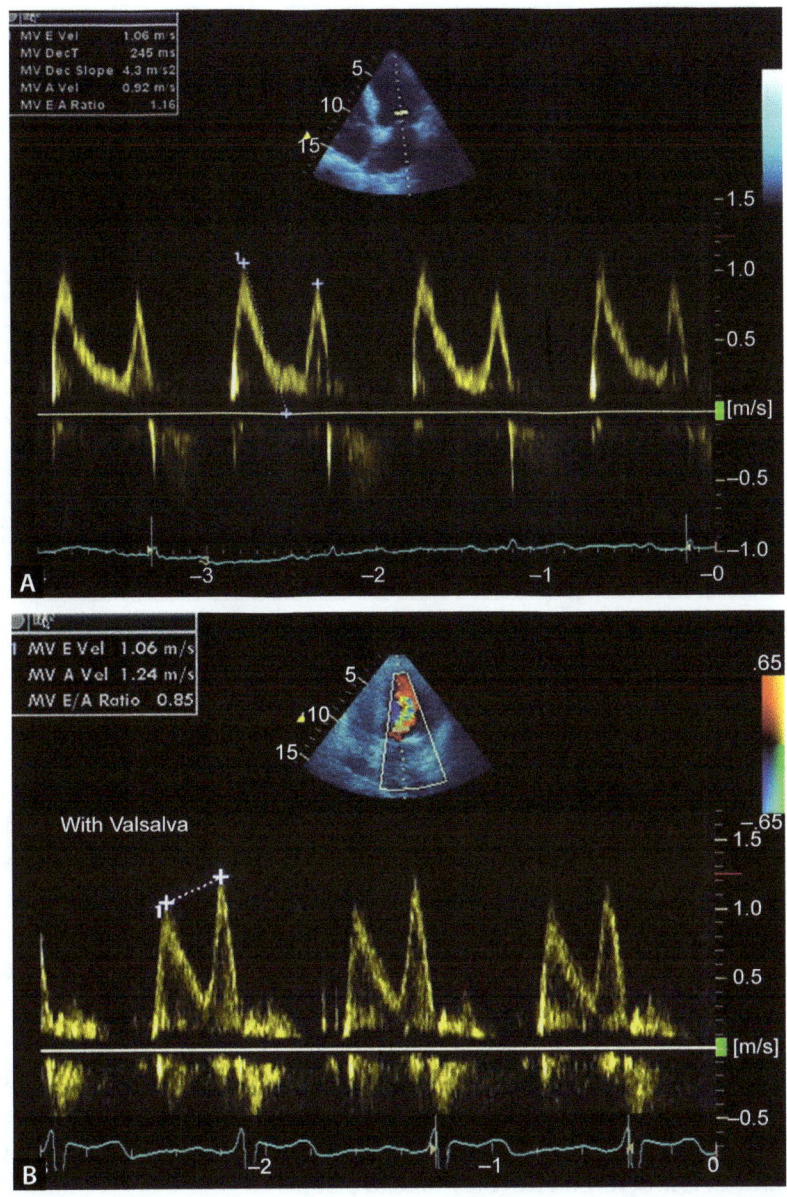

Figs. 5.26A and B: (A) Pseudonormal pattern grade-II dysfunction; (B) Unmasking pseudonormal with valsalva.

will be more than or equal to 2. In severe forms, the A wave may be so small as to be nearly invisible, and the E/A ratio may reach very high values of 5 or more.

When filling pressures are high, flow into the ventricle will start early and filling will terminate quickly. Therefore, typical additional signs of restrictive filling include a short IVRT (≤70 ms) and DT (<140 ms) (Fig. 5.27).

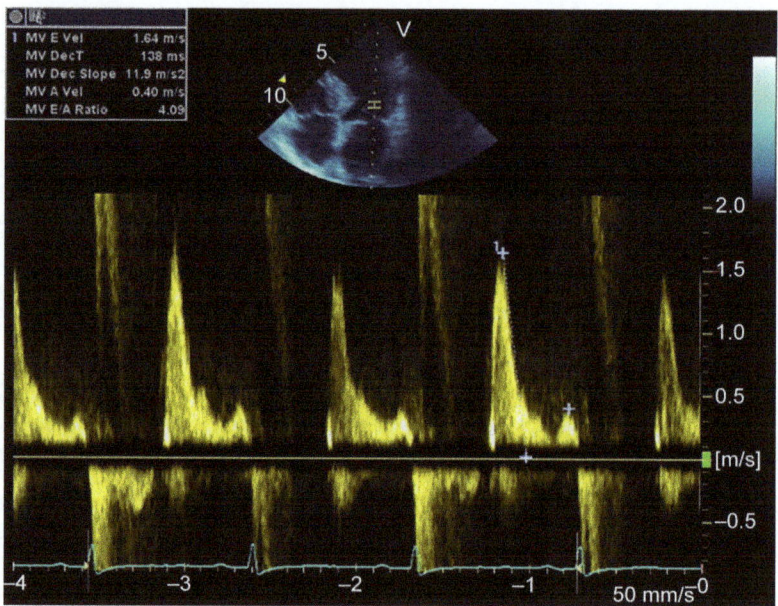

Fig. 5.27: Restrictive picture—grade-III diastolic dysfunction.

Tissue Doppler Imaging of Mitral Valve Annulus

The motion of the MV annulus mirrors systolic as well as diastolic events. During systole, the annulus moves caudally toward the apex; and during diastole, it moves cranially toward the atrium. The motion of the annulus can be recorded with the help of PW TDI at the medial (septal) as well as the lateral ring (in a 4-chamber view).

The tracing of the Doppler wave is a mirror image of negative deflection of diastolic waves same as MV inflow. Except that, they are called as e'(e prime) and a'(a prime). Together with the MV inflow Doppler that complete the diagnostics of diastolic dysfunction.

A ratio of E/e' helps in understanding the filling pressures and diastolic dysfunction. A ratio more than 15 correlates with high LV filling pressures and presence of diastolic dysfunction. A ratio of less than 8 correlates with normal filling pressures and no diastolic dysfunction. Between 8 and 15 is indeterminate (Figs. 5.28 to 5.30).

By comparing all the modalities together one can determine the degree of diastolic dysfunction (Fig. 5.31). A similar assessment can be made using pulmonary valve inflow as well as color Doppler with M mode. However, there are some indirect signs of diastolic dysfunction, which can help to guide toward diastolic dysfunction like presence of LV wall hypertrophy or increased filling pressures as seen by bulge of interatrial septum toward right and dilated pulmonary veins.

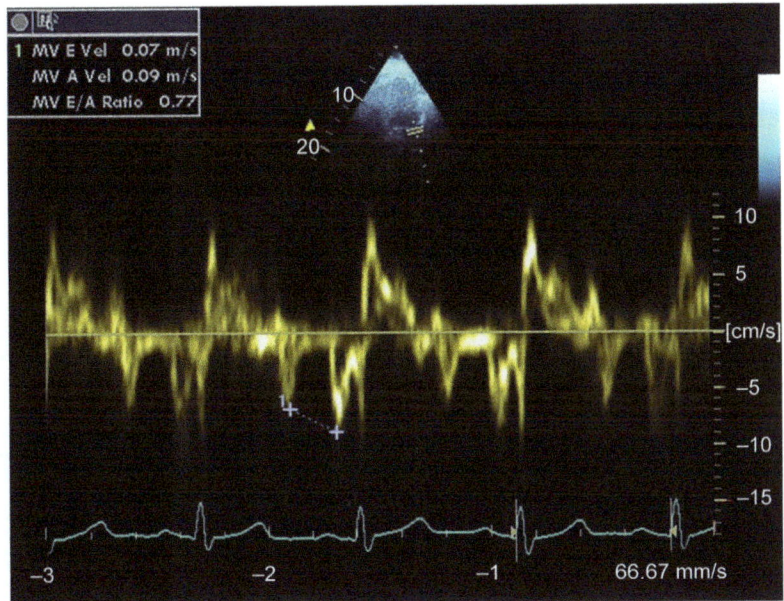

Fig. 5.28: Abnormal relaxation.

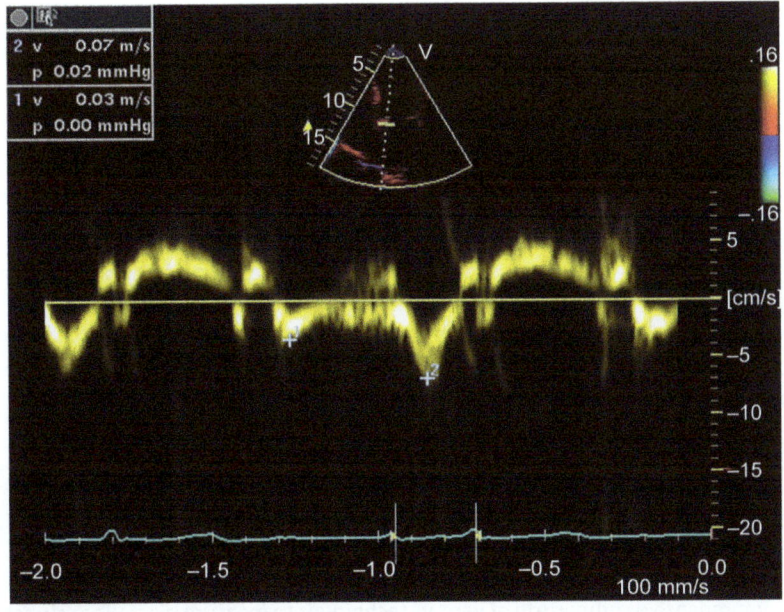

Fig. 5.29: Pseudonormal.

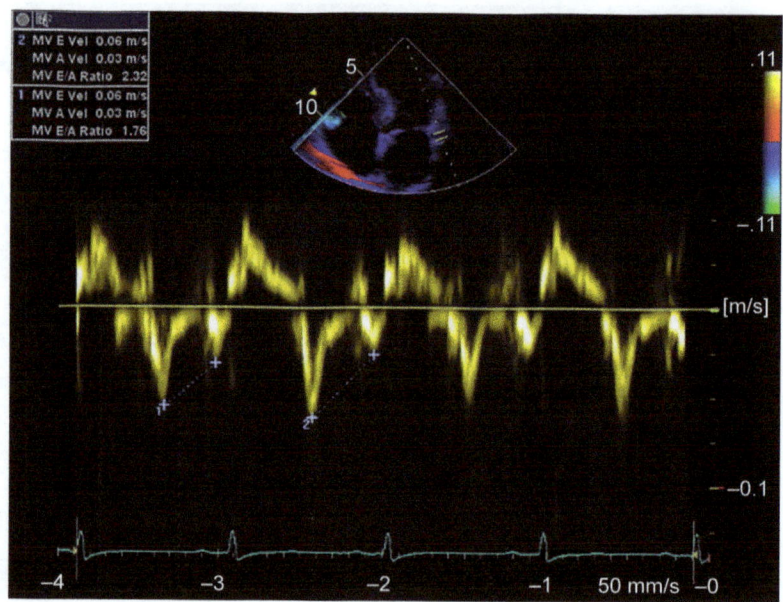

Fig. 5.30: Restrictive pattern.

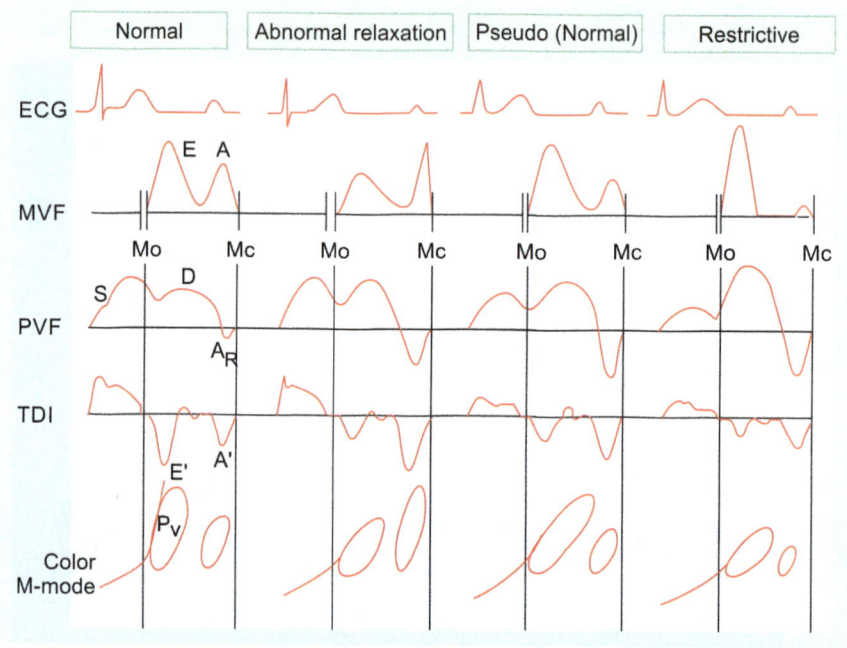

Fig. 5.31: A comprehensive comparison of various techniques to measure diastolic dysfunction. (ECG: electrocardiography; MVF: mitral flow; PVF: pulmonary venous flow; TDI: tissue Doppler).

REFERENCES

1. Patterson SW, Starling EH. On the mechanical factors which determine the output of the ventricles. J Physiol. 1914;48:357-79.
2. Guyton ACJC, Coleman TG. Circulatory Physiology: Cardiac Output and its Regulation. Philadelphia, PA: Saunders; 1973.
3. Wiedemann HP, Wheeler AP, Bernard GR, et al. Comparison of two fluid-management strategies in acute lung injury. N Engl J Med. 2006;354:2564-75.
4. Bagshaw SM, Brophy PD, Cruz D, et al. Fluid balance as a biomarker: impact of fluid overload on outcome in critically ill patients with acute kidney injury. Crit Care. 2008;12:169.
5. Kanji HD, McCallum J, Sirounis D, et al. Limited echocardiography-guided therapy in subacute shock is associated with change in management and improved outcomes. J Crit Care. 2014;29:700-5.
6. Brennan JM, Blair JE, Goonewardena S, et al. Reappraisal of the use of inferior vena cava for estimating right atrial pressure. J Am Soc Echocardiogr. 2007;20:857-61.
7. Brennan JM, Ronan A, Goonewardena S, et al. Handcarried ultrasound measurement of the inferior vena cava for assessment of intravascular volume status in the outpatient hemodialysis clinic. Clin J Am Soc Nephrol. 2006;1:749-53.
8. Goonewardena SN, Gemignani A, Ronan A, et al. Comparison of hand-carried ultrasound assessment of the inferior vena cava and N-terminal pro-brain natriuretic peptide for predicting readmission after hospitalization for acute decompensated heart failure. JACC Cardiovasc Imag. 2008;1:595-601.
9. Lang RM, Badano LP, Mor-Avi V, et al. Recommendations for cardiac chamber quantification by echocardiography in adults: an update from the American Society of Echocardiography and the European Association of Cardiovascular Imaging. J Am Soc Echocardiogr. 2015;28:1-39.e14.
10. Porter TR, Shillcutt SK, Adams MS, et al. Guidelines for the use of echocardiography as a monitor for therapeutic intervention in adults: a report from the American Society of Echocardiography. J Am Soc Echocardiogr. 2015;28:40-56.
11. Spencer KT, Kimura BJ, Korcarz CE, et al. Focused cardiac ultrasound: recommendations from the American Society of Echocardiography. J Am Soc Echocardiogr. 2013;26:567-81.
12. Cherpanath TG, Hirsch A, Geerts BF, et al. Predicting fluid responsiveness by passive leg raising: a systematic review and meta-analysis of 23 clinical trials. Crit Care Med. 2016;44:981-91.
13. Monnet X, Rienzo M, Osman D, et al. Passive leg raising predicts fluid responsiveness in the critically ill. Crit Care Med. 2006;34:1402-7.
14. Cherpanath TG, Hirsch A, Geerts BF, et al. Predicting fluid responsiveness by passive leg raising: a systematic review and meta-analysis of 23 clinical trials. Crit Care Med. 2016;44:981-91.
15. Mahjoub Y, Touzeau J, Airapetian N, et al. The passive leg-raising maneuver cannot accurately predict fluid responsiveness in patients with intra-abdominal hypertension. Crit Care Med. 2010;38:1824-9.
16. Mahjoub Y, Pila C, Friggeri A, et al. Assessing fluid responsiveness in critically ill patients: false-positive pulse pressure variation is detected by Doppler echocardiographic evaluation of the right ventricle. Crit Care Med. 2009;37:2570-5.
17. Barbier C, Loubieres Y, Schmit C, et al. Respiratory changes in inferior vena cava diameter are helpful in predicting fluid responsiveness in ventilated septic patients. Intensive Care Med. 2004;30:1740-6.
18. Charbonneau H, Riu B, Faron M, et al. Predicting preload responsiveness using simultaneous recordings of inferior and superior vena cavae diameters. Crit Care. 2014;18:473.
19. Feissel M, Michard F, Faller JP, et al. The respiratory variation in inferior vena cava diameter as a guide to fluid therapy. Intensive Care Med. 2004;30:1834-7.

20. Machare-Delgado E, Decaro M, Marik PE. Inferior vena cava variation compared to pulse contour analysis as predictors of fluid responsiveness: a prospective cohort study. J Intensive Care Med. 2011;26:116-24.
21. Via G, Tavazzi G, Price S. Ten situations where inferior vena cava ultrasound may fail to accurately predict fluid responsiveness: a physiologically based point of view. Intensive Care Med. 2016;42:1164-7.
22. Gignon L, Roger C, Bastide S, et al. Influence of diaphragmatic motion on inferior vena cava diameter respiratory variations in healthy volunteers. Anesthesiology. 2016;124:1338-46.
23. Airapetian N, Maizel J, Alyamani O, et al. Does inferior vena cava respiratory variability predict fluid responsiveness in spontaneously breathing patients? Crit Care. 2015;19:400.
24. Via G, Tavazzi G, Price S. Ten situations where inferior vena cava ultrasound may fail to accurately predict fluid responsiveness: a physiologically based point of view. Intensive Care Med. 2016;42:1164-7.
25. Reuter DA, Felbinger TW, Schmidt C, et al. Stroke volume variations for the assessment of cardiac responsiveness to volume loading in mechanically ventilated patients. Intensive Care Med. 2002;28:392-8.
26. Feissel M, Michard F, Mangin I, et al. Respiratory changes in aortic blood velocity as an indicator of fluid responsiveness in patients with septic shock. Chest. 2001;119:867-73.
27. Rex S, Brose S, Metzelder S, et al. Prediction of fluid responsiveness during cardiac surgery. Br J Anesth. 2004;93:782-8.
28. Broch O, Renner J, Gruenewald M, et al. Variation of left ventricular outflow tract velocity and global end-diastolic volume index reliably predict fluid responsiveness in cardiac surgery patients. J Crit Care. 2012;27:325.e7-13.
29. Melamed R, Sprenkle MD, Ulstad VK, et al. Assessment of left ventricular function by intensivists using hand-held echocardiography. Chest. 2009;135:1416-20.
30. Slama M, Maizel J. Echocardiographic measurement of ventricular function. Curr Opin Crit Care. 2006;12:241-8.
31. Vieillard-Baron A, Prin S, Chergui K, et al. Echo-Doppler demonstration of acute cor pulmonale at the bedside in the medical intensive care unit. Am J Respir Crit Care Med. 2002;166:1310-9.
32. Goldhaber SZ. Echocardiography in the management of pulmonary embolism. Ann Intern Med. 2002;136:691-70.
33. Rudski LG, Lai WW, Afilalo J, et al. Guidelines for the echocardiographic assessment of the right heart in adults: A report from the American Society of Echocardiography. J Am Soc Echocardiogr. 2010;23:685-713.
34. Chambers JB. Clinical echocardiography. London: BMJ Publishing Group; 1995.
35. Feigenbaum H. Echocardiography, 1st edition. Philadelphia: Lea and Febiger; 1972.
36. Kaddoura S. Echo made easy, 3rd edition. London: Elsevier; 2016.

CHAPTER

Abdominal Aortic Aneurysm, Deep Vein Thrombosis and Pulmonary Embolism: Use of Ultrasound

Srishti Jain, Ravindra Zore

ABDOMINAL AORTIC ANEURYSM

Ruptured abdominal aortic aneurysm (AAA) is potentially a fatal condition with increasing prevalence in elderly population. AAA is misdiagnosed many times as very few patients present with classical symptoms like abdominal or flank pain, shock and pulsatile abdominal mass. If it is not diagnosed early, AAA can have catastrophic results. In patients with suspected ruptured aneurysm, ultrasound can provide rapid diagnosis and thus prevent unnecessary computed tomography (CT) and facilitate urgent surgery if required.[1]

SCANNING OF ABDOMINAL AORTA

Curvilinear probe with frequency of 1–5 MHz is used as it provides better penetration. Probe is applied in abdominal orientation with marker to the right of patient. Abdominal aorta gives rise to celiac trunk, superior mesenteric artery (SMA) and renal arteries in succession after entering below diaphragm. Most of AAA arises distal to origin of renal arteries. With patient in supine position, abdominal aorta is scanned in transverse plane from epigastrium till bifurcation of aorta into iliac arteries. It has anechoic lumen with echogenic walls. Aorta is identified to the left of midline and inferior vena cava (IVC) to the right against vertebral column (Fig. 6.1). Gentle pressure can be applied to dispel bowel gas for better visualization of aorta. For longitudinal view, probe is rotated through 90° so marker is pointed towards head of the patient.

ABDOMINAL AORTIC DIAMETER

Diameter of aorta should be measured in longitudinal as well as in transverse section from outer wall to outer wall. In young males normal aortic diameter at infra-renal level is approximately 2.3 cm and in females it is 1.9 cm. Diagnosis of AAA include:
- Focal dilatation of AA more than 3 cm.
- Increase in aortic diameter to 1.5 times the normal diameter.

In case of aneurysm, shape and location must be noted. Also maximum true length and diameter of aneurysm should be measured. Aneurysmal sac should be measured from outer wall

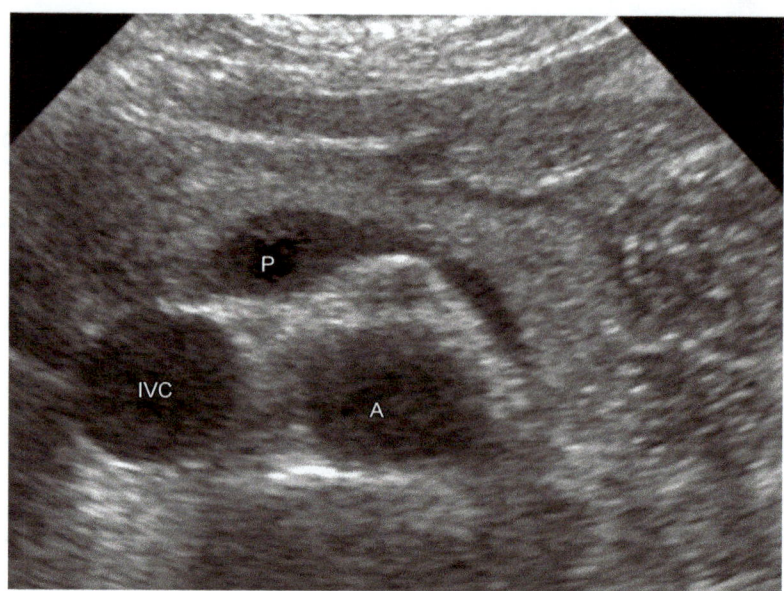

Fig. 6.1: Transverse section showing normal appearance of abdominal aorta (A: abdominal aorta; IVC: inferior vena cava; P: portal vein).[2]

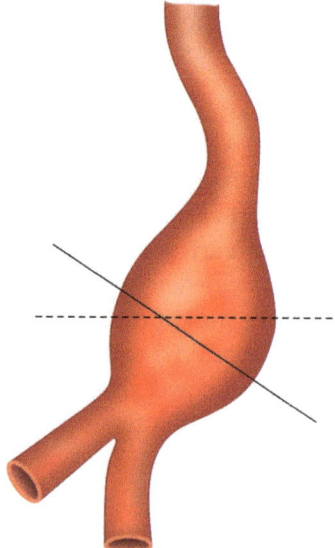

Fig. 6.2: The correct method of measuring an abdominal aortic aneurysm (AAA) is perpendicular to the long-axis of the aorta as shown by the continuous line.[2]

to outer wall in longitudinal section. Diameter should be measured in transverse section perpendicular to long axis of aorta especially in ectatic aneurysms where transverse measurement may not represent true diameter as it is actually oblique measurement (Figs. 6.2 and 6.3).[2]

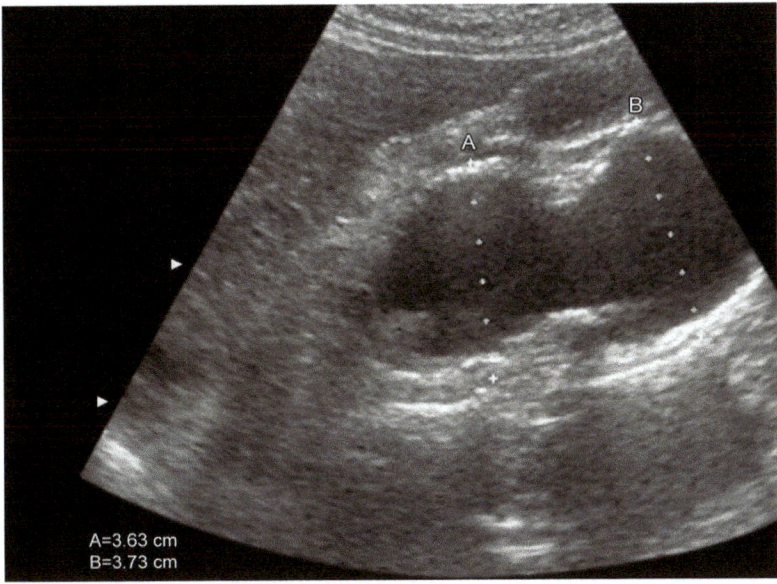

Fig. 6.3: Longitudinal section of aorta showing aneurysm.[2]

ABDOMINAL AORTIC DISSECTION

Abdominal aortic dissection is mainly seen in older population mainly affecting 60–70 years. Hypertension is the major-risk factor. Abdominal aortic dissection is usually seen with involvement of thoracic aorta also.

On ultrasound, it is diagnosed with presence intimal flap which is seen as linear hyperechoic area within lumen of aorta. It divides aortic lumen into true and false lumen.[2]

LIMITATIONS OF AORTIC SONOGRAPHY[2]

- Obesity and bowel gas are two major hurdles for abdominal scan.
- Small aneurysms can be missed.
- True aortic or aneurysm diameter can be exaggerated due to angled measurements as explained earlier.
- Retroperitoneal hemorrhage due to rupture AAA can be overlooked.
- Mural thrombi can mimic aortic dissection due to echogenicities giving rise to appearance of two lumens within aorta.

DEEP VEIN THROMBOSIS

Venous thromboembolism as a condition includes deep vein thrombosis (DVT) to pulmonary embolism (PE) in continuum. PE can manifest in approximately 50% of patients with DVT. Lower limb DVT contributes to around 90% of cases of PE and they mostly originate from proximal veins like common femoral, superficial femoral and popliteal veins. Bedside ultrasound is an excellent tool for screening of DVT and PE since it has sensitivity and specificity is more than 95% for both upper limb and proximal lower limb DVT. Also it is noninvasive, fast, easily reproducible and cost-effective modality.[3]

LOWER LIMB VENOUS ULTRASOUND

A linear array probe with frequency of 5–10 MHz is used for lower limb venous examination. Ultrasound is performed with probe marker towards patient's right side. Two characteristic findings of DVT on ultrasound include non-compressibility of vein and/or visualization of thrombus. When thrombus is visualized, compression test is not performed as it may dislodge thrombus. Longitudinal view can be used to confirm echogenic material as thrombus.[4]

FEMORAL VEIN

For femoral vein ultrasound patient should be in supine position with the hip externally rotated and flexed (Fig. 6.4). The linear probe is placed in the transverse position at the level of the inguinal ligament with the probe marker pointed towards the patient's right. Here femoral vein will be seen medial to femoral artery (Fig. 6.5). Compression test is performed. Once compressibility of both the deep and superficial femoral veins is confirmed, the examination may move on to the popliteal vein.

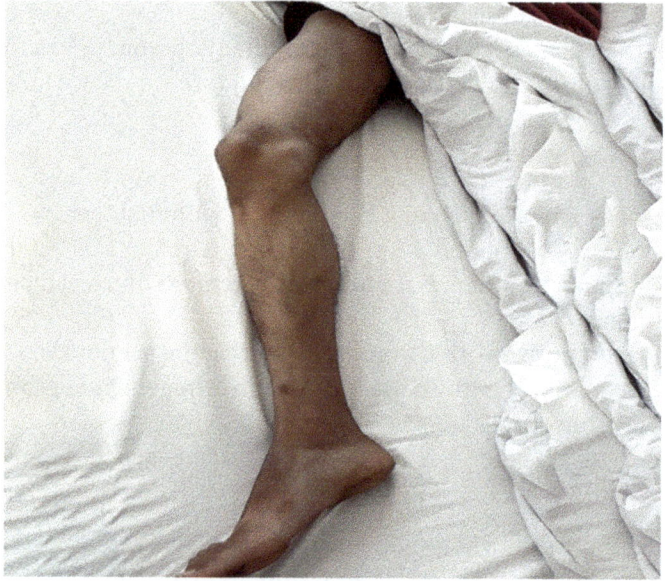

Fig. 6.4: Position for scanning femoral vein.

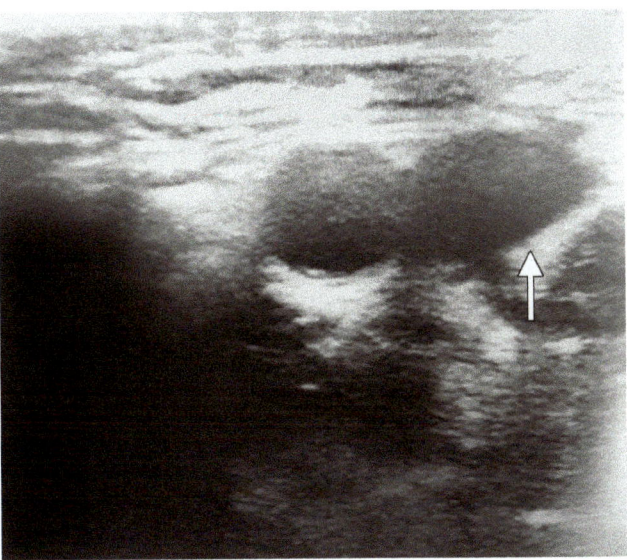

Fig. 6.5: Right femoral vein (arrow) with femoral artery lateral.

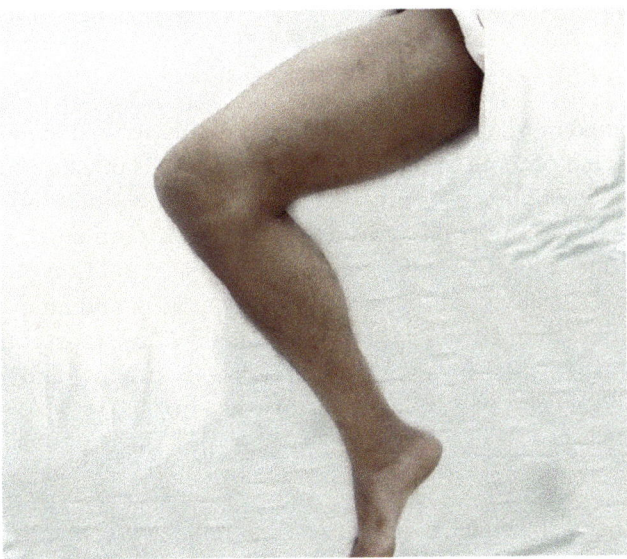

Fig. 6.6: Showing position for scanning popliteal vein.

POPLITEAL VEIN

For popliteal vein examination knee should be flexed at 45° and externally rotated (Fig. 6.6). In popliteal fossa vein is posterior to artery. Due to the posterior approach of probe, popliteal vein appears superficial to artery and near to skin. Compression test is performed from distal 2 cm of popliteal vein up to its proximal part of trifurcation into calf veins (Fig. 6.7).[4]

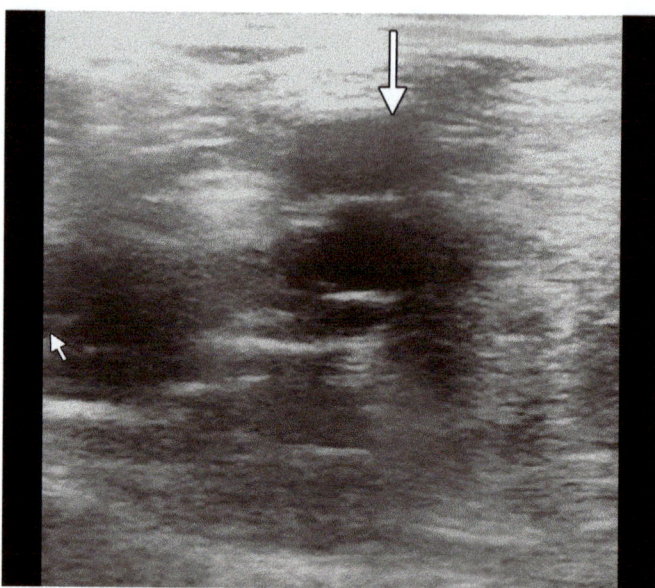

Fig. 6.7: Popliteal vein (arrow) with popliteal artery below.

COMPRESSION TEST

This test is performed in transverse plane and pressure is applied in perpendicular direction. As pressure is applied on both anterior and posterior walls of vein should be approximated and lumen should be obliterated. Sufficient amount of pressure is indicated by deformation of adjacent artery (Fig. 6.8). If vein does not collapse with pressure causing deformation of artery then it indicates presence of thrombus in vein (Fig. 6.9).[4] Compression-only studies for proximal DVT have sensitivity of 100%, a specificity of 98%, and an overall accuracy of 99%. There are various ultrasound protocols for diagnosing DVT but most commonly applied is two region compression test which involves femoral veins 1–2 cm above and below saphenofemoral junction and popliteal veins up to confluence of calf vein.[5]

PITFALLS

- An artery can be mistaken for noncompressible vein leading to misdiagnosis of DVT.
- Inguinal lymphadenopathy can be mistaken for noncompressible common femoral vein.
    - On longitudinal scan lymph nodes have definite extent and also they are superficial compared to vein.
- Pulmonary embolism cannot be ruled out even with negative scan for lower limb DVT.

PULMONARY EMBOLISM

Pulmonary embolism (PE) is serious complication of VTE and carries high mortality rate. PE can present with breathlessness, chest pain, hypotension or syncope associated with tachycardia, tachypnea and hypotension.[3] Pulmonary angiography is the gold standard

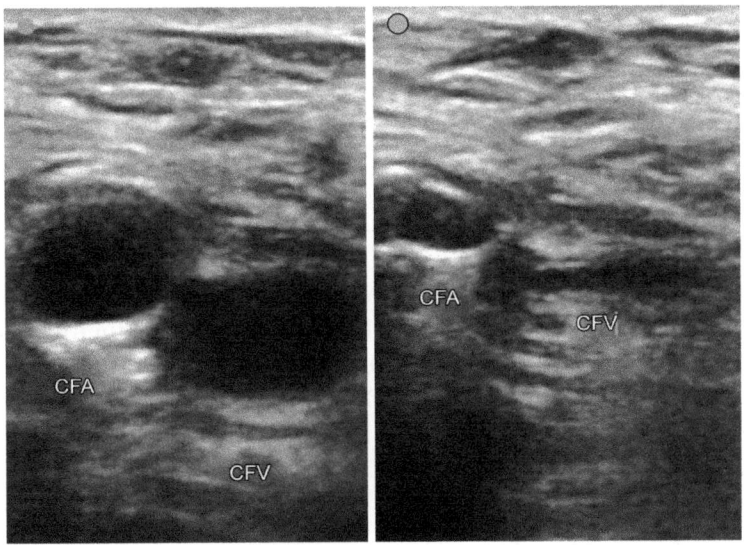

Fig. 6.8: On right side showing normal compression test with complete obliteration of lumen.[4]
CFA: Common femoral artery; CFV: common femoral vein.

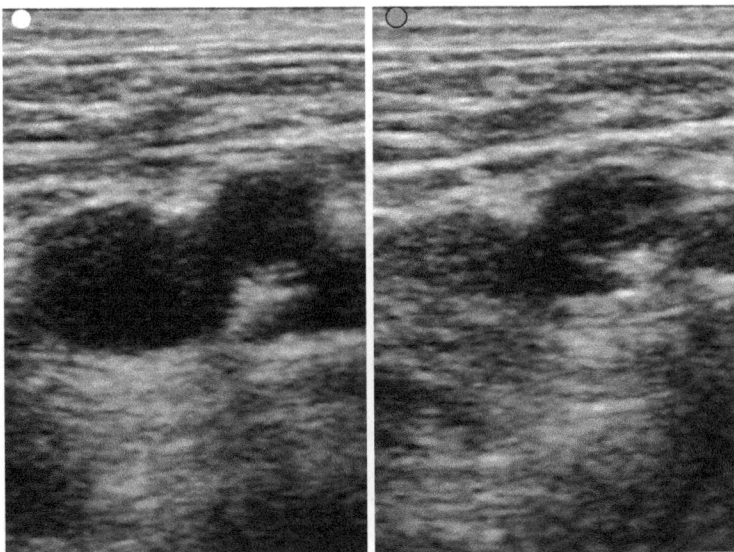

Fig. 6.9: Positive compression: On the right showing echogenic material in the vessel lumen with loss of collapsibility.[6]

for diagnosis of PE but CT chest with angiography is the most-widely used imaging method. Echocardiography is important not only for diagnosis of PE but it has therapeutic implications also. In hemodynamically unstable patients with suspected PE, echocardiography can be used to rule out PE as a cause of hypotension. Patient can undergo reperfusion therapy based on echocardiography diagnosis if CT is not feasible due to hemodynamic unstable condition.[6]

ECHOCARDIOGRAPHIC FINDINGS IN PULMONARY EMBOLISM[6]

- Right ventricular dilatation.
- Right ventricular hypokinesia.
- Abnormal septal position and paradoxical systolic motion.
- Thromboemboli within the right heart or pulmonary artery.

Right Ventricular Dilatation

Right ventricle (RV) is best examined in apical 4-chamber view and measurements are carried out in end diastole. RV dilatation is indicated by diameter is greater than 42 mm at the base and greater than 35 mm at midlevel. Also if longitudinal dimensions are greater than 86 mm then it suggests RV enlargement. With eyeballing if RV appears significantly larger than left ventricle (LV) in spite of normal dimensions, it can be labeled as dilated RV (Fig. 6.10).[7]

Right Ventricular Hypokinesis

Right ventricular free wall hypokinesia is present with preserved apical contractility which is also known as McConnell's sign (Fig. 6.11). It helps to diagnose RV dysfunction due to PE even with preexisting cardiorespiratory conditions.[6] In massive PE is greater than 90% patients will have McConnell's sign present.[8]

Abnormal Septal Position and Paradoxical Motion

This is better appreciated in parasternal short-axis and apical 4 chamber view. Due to acute pulmonary hypertension interventricular septum becomes flat giving rise to *D* shaped LV.

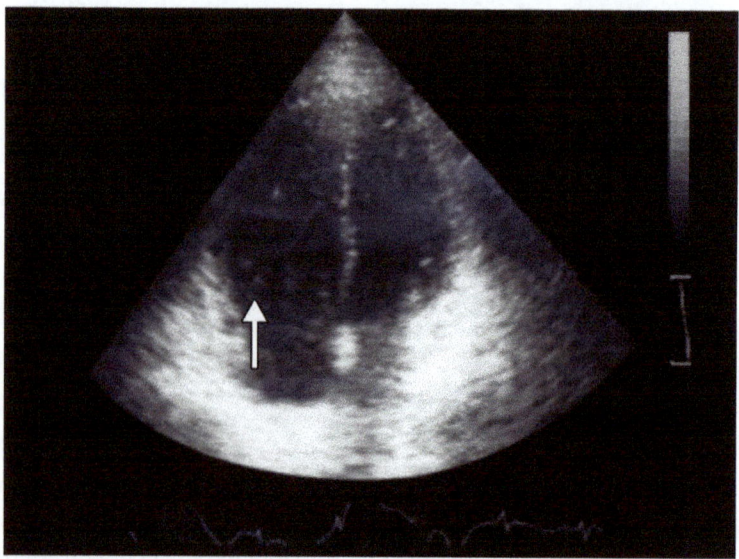

Fig. 6.10: Right ventricular dilatation in apical view (arrow).[8]

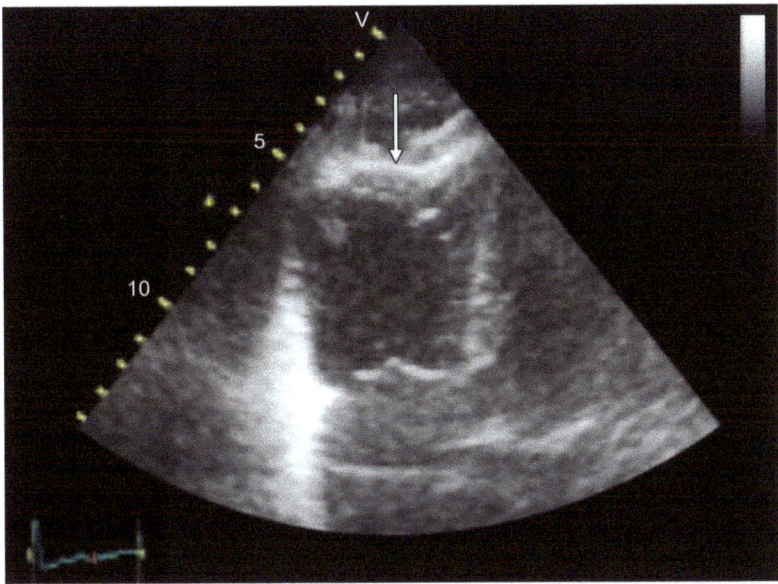

Fig. 6.11: Right ventricle free wall hypokinesia with apical sparing (arrow)[9] known as McConnell's sign.

Interventricular septum can show paradoxical motion with bulging into LV cavity as RV continues to contract in end systole even after LV relaxes. This occurs as LV does not get time to adapt to development of acute pulmonary hypertension. These features help to distinguish between acute and chronic PHT.[8]

Thromboemboli Within Right Side Heart or Pulmonary Artery

Only 18% of patients in critical care setting show presence of thrombus in right heart on echocardiography. Their presence confirms diagnosis of PE and indicates severe RV dysfunction with poor prognosis.[6]

LUNG ULTRASOUND IN PULMONARY EMBOLISM

Any patient presenting with dyspnea, Beside Lung Ultrasound in Emergency (BLUE) protocol is applied for lung examination.[10] Lung ultrasound is supportive tool for diagnosing PE especially in hemodynamically unstable patients. It may show peripheral consolidation pattern due to embolic occlusion.

LOWER LIMB COMPRESSION ULTRASOUND

Incomplete compressibility of vein indicates presence of thrombus and is sufficient for diagnosis of DVT. For symptomatic DVT, it has sensitivity greater than 90% and specificity approximately 95%. In suspected PE, finding of DVT is considered enough to start with anticoagulant therapy without further evaluation.[6]

SUMMARY

Thus any patient presenting with shock, diagnosis can be achieved by performing bedside ultrasound. Any patient presenting with shock can be examined by RUSH (Rapid Ultrasound in Shock) protocol which has pump (heart), tank (lung) and pipes (aorta, IVC and lower limb veins) components. It may show leaking pipes as in ruptured AAA as a cause of hypovolemic shock. On the other hand, it can diagnose PE as a cause of obstructive shock with depressed pump (RV dysfunction), and obstructed pipes (DVT in lower limb veins).[10]

REFERENCES

1. Kuhn M, Bonnin RL, Davey MJ, Rowland JL, et al. Emergency department ultrasound scanning for abdominal aortic aneurysm: accessible, accurate, and advantageous. Ann Emerg Med. 2000; 36: 219-23.
2. Bhatt S, Ghazale H, Dogra VS. Sonographic evaluation of the abdominal aorta. Ultrasound Clinics 2. 2007; 437-53.
3. Fox JC, Bertoglio KC. Emergency Physician Performed Ultrasound for DVT Evaluation. Thrombosis Vol. 2011; Article ID 938709: 4 pages.
4. DiBello C, Koenig S. Diagnosis of deep venous thrombosis by critical care physicians using compression ultrasound. The Open Critical Care Medicine Journal 2010; 3: 43-7.
5. Lewiss RE, Kaban NL, Saul T. Point-of-care ultrasound for a deep venous thrombosis. Global Heart December 2013; 8(4):329-33.
6. Konstantinides SV, Torbicki A, Agnelli G, et al. 2014 ESC Guidelines on the diagnosis and management of acute pulmonary embolism. The Task Force for the Diagnosis and Management of Acute Pulmonary Embolism of the European Society of Cardiology (ESC). European Heart Journal 2014; 35: 3033–80.
7. Rudski LG, Lai WW, Afilalo J, et al. Guidelines for the Echocardiographic Assessment of the Right Heart in Adults: A Report from the American Society of Echocardiography Endorsed by the European Association of Echocardiography, a registered branch of the European Society of Cardiology, and the Canadian Society of Echocardiography. J Am Soc Echocardiography 2010; 23: 685-713.
8. Cohen R, Loarte P, Navarro V, et al. Echocardiographic findings in pulmonary embolism: An important guide for the management of the patient. World Journal of Cardiovascular Diseases 2012; 2: 161-4.
9. Shafiq Q, Assaly R, Kanjwal Y. Case Report—McConnell Sign in a Patient with Massive Acute Pulmonary Embolism. Case Reports in Cardiology Volume 2011; Article ID 201097: 3 pages.
10. Seif D, Perera P, Mailhot T, et al. Bedside ultrasound in resuscitation and the rapid ultrasound in shock protocol. Critical Care Research and Practice. Volume 2012; Article ID 503254:14 pages.

Ultrasound of the Gallbladder, Pancreas and Bowel in Emergencies

Pratibha Patel

INTRODUCTION

Gallbladder

Gallbladder pathology can develop in intensive care unit (ICU) patients in completely unrelated conditions, and can result in significant morbidity and mortality in already critically ill patients.

CONDITIONS

- Cholelithiasis (gall stones)
- Choledocholithiasis
- Cholecystitis:
  – Calculous
  – Acalculous

ANATOMY

Gallbladder (GB) lies in a fossa below liver between right and quadrate lobe called as GB fossa. It has a neck body and fundus.

The GB fundus is seen as globular projection below liver its position and shape varies as per the fasting status, volume and anatomy. Body is continuation of fundus and towards the upper end body narrows and that is the neck which continues as into cystic duct, it lies in a constant position to portal vein.

Its transverse diameter is around 4 cm if it is greater than 4 cm it signifies distended.
Capacity of gallbladder: 50 mL

Common Bile Duct

It is formed by union of hepatic duct and cystic duct. Its normal diameter is around 6 mm or less.

Ultrasound

- Probe 3.5–5.0 curvilinear or abdominal probe.
- *Patient's position*: Supine or left lateral decubitus.
- Fasting status is preferred as GB contracts after meals.

Probe Placement

Longitudinal view: Place the probe subcostal or below costal margins with probe marker pointing cephalic towards midaxillary line. Identify the landmarks diaphragm as bright hyperechoic line liver and kidney now angle the probe slightly caudal and ask patient to take deep breath for better view of GB (Figs. 7.1 and 7.2).

Transverse view: Same position but probe marker towards right side or place probe medially in subcostal region and sweep down laterally. This view is better to see GB and CBD.

Normal: GB appears as a saccular fluid-filled structure.

Landmark

Undivided right portal vein: Align the probe angle along the imaginary line between axilla and umbilicus in subcostal position.

Main lobar fissure seen as bright hyperechoic line extending from right portal vein to GB Fossa.

- Image GB in sagittal and transverse section
- *Take volume measurement*: Length × breadth × width

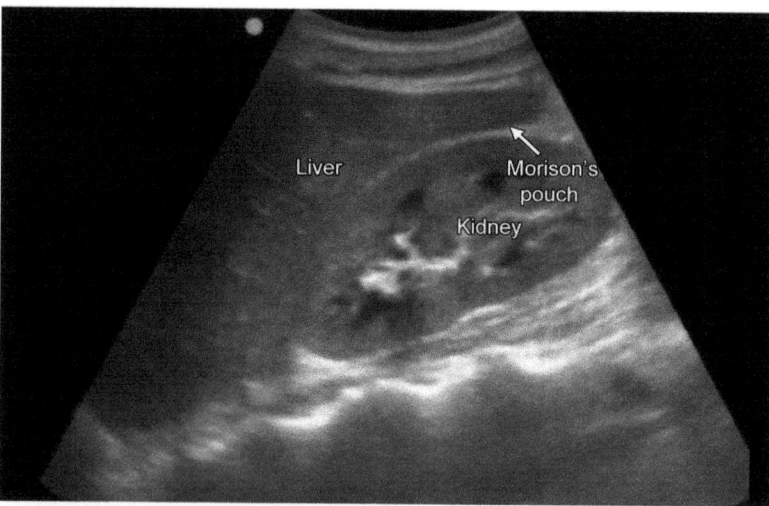

Fig. 7.1: Right upper quadrant view: diaphragm, liver and right kidney.

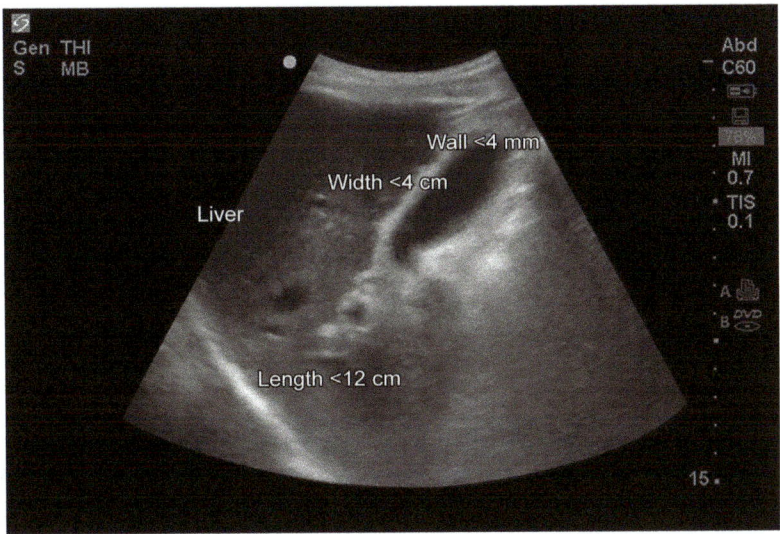

Fig. 7.2: Gallbladder: dimensions.

- Measure GB wall thickness in lateral mid position
- Try to visualize CBD, pancreas and liver.

Gallbladder can be confused with bowel. Scan GB in longitudinal and transverse planes GB will show narrow neck towards cystic duct.

FINDINGS AND CONDITIONS

- *Murphy's sign:* It is elicited presence of pain by application of pressure by probe over GB fundus.
  Pain suggests cholecystitis or cholelithiasis pain may be absent in acalculous cholecystitis.
- *Gallbladder distension:* It is said to be distended if it is greater than 10 cm in length and breadth greater than 4 cm in transverse plane. It includes:
  - It indicates delayed emptying.
  - Functional or mechanical obstruction of cystic duct.
  - Cause—cholecystitis.
- Gallbladder calculi:
  - Appears as highly-reflective echoes with posterior acoustic shadows.
  - Varied appearance according to composition of stone.
  - All stones must move with change in position and produce shadows.
  - Echoes which do not cast shadows represent sludge.
- Gallbladder wall thickening:
  - Normal wall measures about 3 mm or less.
  - Thickened wall appears as two echogenic lines with hypoechoic region between them — suggesting inflammation and/or edema.

- Non-fasting GB wall also appears thickened because of contraction.
- *Conditions:* Calculous cholecystitis, acalculous cholecystitis and tropical fever as dengue. Sometimes in inflammatory conditions of abdomen:
  - *Acalculous cholecystitis:* More common in critical care settings (0.2–10%). 40–100% of cases are advanced with gangrene, empyema or perforation which carries a grave prognosis. Hence diagnosis in time is of great importance.
- Pericholecystic fluid:
  - Fluid around gallbladder.
  - May be confused with ascites.
- Air in gallbladder lumen or wall:
  - Seen as hyperechoic shadow in lumen.
  - *Condition:* Emphysematous cholecystitis—a surgical emergency.
  - Seen in acute cholecystitis (mainly in GB perforation).
  - Pancreatitis.

Common Bile Duct

It runs along and anterior to portal vein. Best place to measure it is at porta hepatis (Fig. 7.3).

Identification of Portal Vein

- Place the probe in subcostal region and change the angle to align it along an imaginary line between axilla and umbilicus. One can see portal vein.

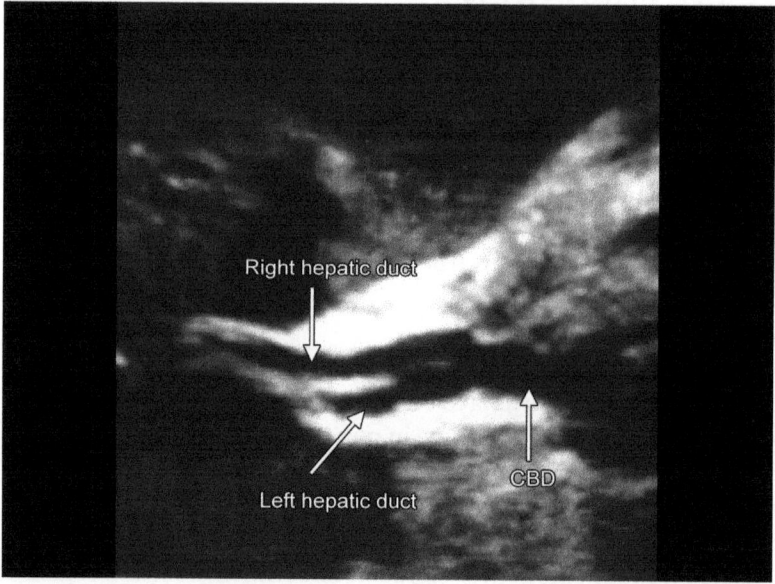

Fig. 7.3: Normal anatomy—common bile duct (CBD).

- Look for GB neck and then portal triad. A large portal vein with its echogenic walls is easy to identify, anterior to inferior vena cava (IVC). The common bile duct (CBD) lies along the front of the portal vein and is smaller caliber and has very echogenic walls (dilated bile duct appears as double channel or parallel channel). The right hepatic artery crosses between the two, hence use of Doppler to distinguish is advised.
- Measure the internal diameter of CBD. Its greatest just at or above the point where hepatic artery crosses between CBD and PV.
- The diameter is greater than 6 mm is suggestive of dilation.
- At times the shape of obstructed end can signify the cause. Tapered end is more consistent with stone and blunt abrupt end with tumor.
- *Conditions:* Migration of gallstones in to CBD is common. USG may not detect actual stones but useful in detecting biliary obstruction which is seen as dilatation of duct.

Other Causes

- Age
- Postcholecystectomy state.

ULTRASOUND OF PANCREAS

- Ultrasound in disease related to pancreas is widely used modality.
- But at times limitations due to obesity and gases in hollow abdominal organs play an important role in poor visualizations. Hence protocols are set up for overcoming this.
- Always tailor your scan to clinical signs and correlate with history.
- *Protocols:* For better visualization.
- Ask patient to take deep inspiration and expirations.
- Ask patient to push the stomach out as if pregnant so that the abdomen is distended against the probe.
- Make patient drink 2–3 glasses of water. This water is used as window to look through when it is in stomach and duodenum. This is called as water load.
- Examining the patient in lateral decubitus and prop-up position may also aid in displacing the gases in stomach and small bowel and colon respectively.
- Fasting for 6 hours is preferred.

Technique

Probe curvilinear or abdominal probe (3.5–5 MHz frequency).

Place the probe high in epigastric region in transverse position with probe marker to right (Fig. 7.4).

Apply pressure on probe gently to displace the bowel gas.

Adjust the image depth (set to grey scale) so that aorta is seen at bottom of the screen (hypoechoic round) above the vertebral margin which is seen as hyperlucent curved bright line.

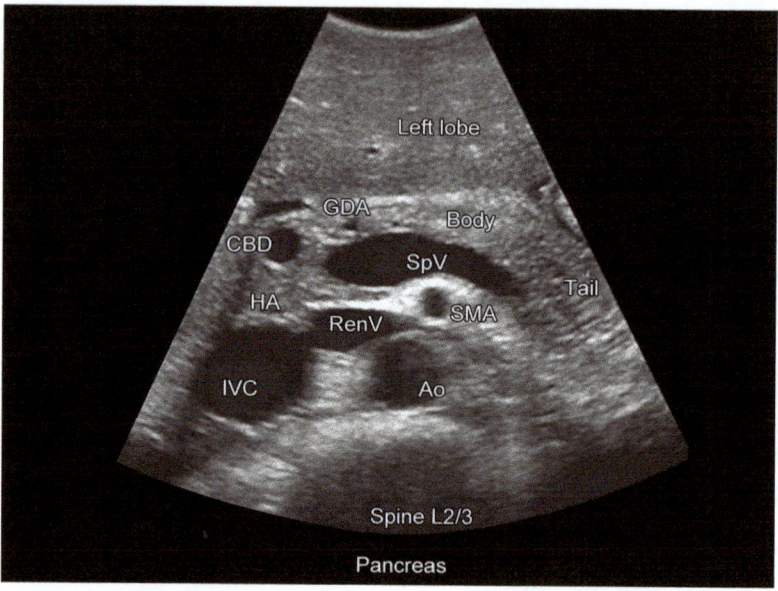

Fig. 7.4: Normal pancreas: transverse view
(CBD: common bile duct; IVC; inferior vena cava; GDA: gastroduodenal artery; SpV: splenic vein; RenV: renal vein; SMA: superior mesenteric artery; Ao: aorta; HA: hepatic artery)

Structures seen are:
- *Head of pancreas:* Scan in both transverse and sagittal planes, as head can be long and continuous, scan left caudally for few centimeters.
- *Body of pancreas*: Scan in transverse. Identify splenic vein (seen at hilum of spleen). Pancreas will be seen superficial to this. Usually both are seen well with transhepatic approach.
- *Tail of pancreas:* Seen in trans-splenic approach.
- Scan transversely, place the heel of probe cephalad and left using spleen as window tail can be seen. Even left intercostal coronal approach can also be used (Fig. 7.5).

ULTRASOUND APPEARANCE

Horse-shoe shaped homogeneous and isoechogenic slightly more echogenic than liver. Peripancreatic fat which is intensely echogenic delineates the margins clearly. Anteriorly stomach and posteriorly splenic vein, superior mesenteric artery and large retroperitoneal aorta and IVC can be seen. If it is hyperechoic that may be due to fatty infiltration.

Normal Measurements

- *Head*: Anteroposterior (AP) diameter around 35 mm.
- *Body*: 10–15 mm.

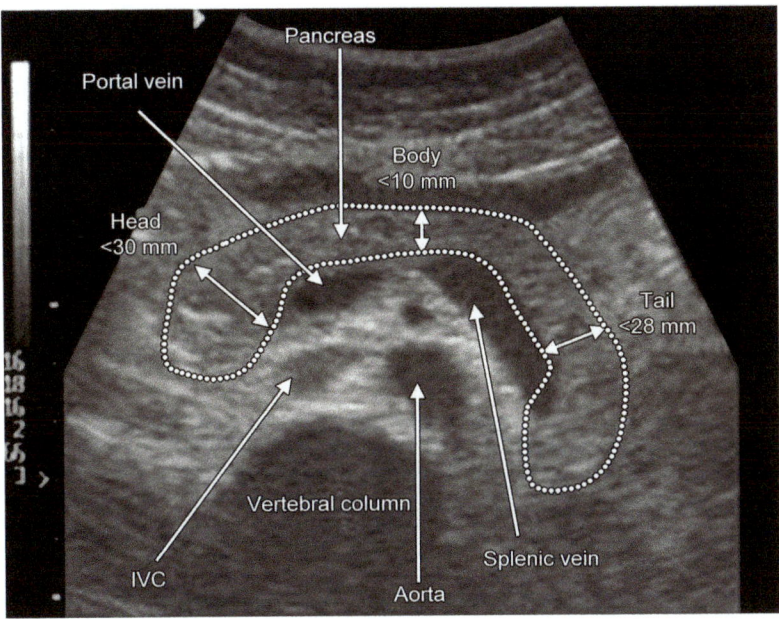

Fig. 7.5: Transverse view of pancreas, parts and normal dimensions (IVC: inferior vena cava)

- *Tail*: 20 mm.
- Duct of Wirsung is seen in middle of organ.
- Examination should be focused on:
    - Pancreatic region:
        * Dimensions.
        * Appearance of parenchyma.
        * Echogenicity.
    - Retroperitoneal region and mesenteric structures for anomalies in blood flow or collections.
    - Recesses for collections and displacement of bowels.

FINDINGS

Acute Pancreatitis

- Increase in volume of pancreas.
- Assessed by displacement of surrounding abdominal organs mainly stomach and transverse colon.
- Quantitatively by measuring AP diameter at level of body of pancreas, if it is more than 24 mm it is associated with increase in volume, signifies edema.
- Parenchyma appears homogeneous (normal) or non-homogeneous.

- Nonhomogenicity correlates with areas of edema and necrosis which may be zonal or confluent.
- In incipient edema pancreatic echoes are normal. In massive edema there is marked hypoechogenicity of pancreas.

Acute Phase

- Identification of peripancreatic collection.
- Areas of necrosis (Fig. 7.6).
- Thrombosis.
- Pseudoaneurysm.
- Superinfection.
- Late phase pseudocyst (Fig. 7.7).
- Segmental portal hypertension syndrome.

Collections

- They appear as hypoechoic or transechoic.
- Margins—recent collections have indefinite or irregular margins.
  - Old collections have clear demarcation.
- Location—peripancreatic is between stomach and pancreas (Fig. 7.8)
  - Distal in peritoneal recess
  - Omental bursa behind stomach

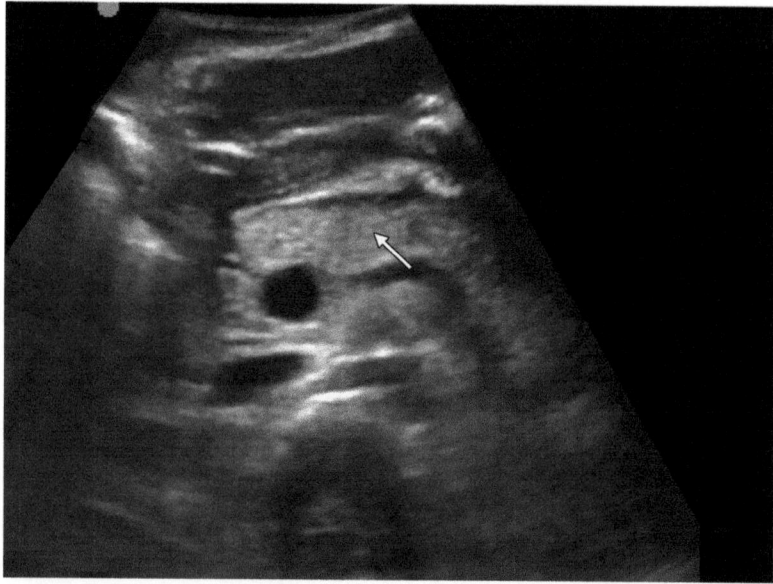

Fig. 7.6: Bulky pancreas and case of pancreatitis.

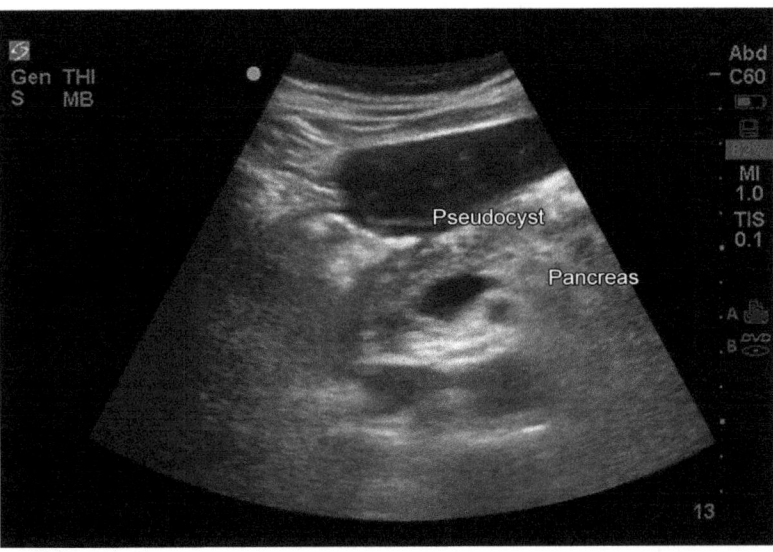
Fig. 7.7: Pancreatic pseudocyst.

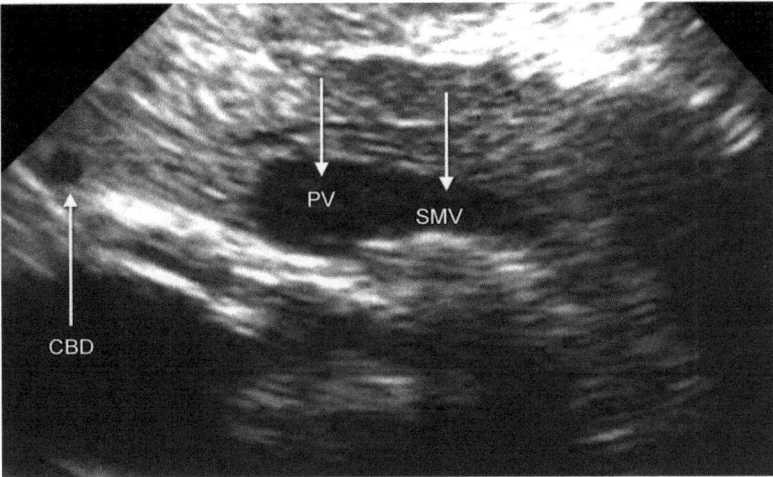
Fig. 7.8: Locating pancreas.
(CBD: common bile duct; PV: portal vein; SMV: superior mesenteric vein).

- In case of large collection it may be in peritoneal cavity amongst intestinal loops or may extend till pouch of Douglas.
- May also be seen in mesentery retroperitoneal or parietocolic groove.
- Enzyme ascites in both pleural recesses is seen as effusions:
  - Echoes may be present in the collections in form of membranes (hematic character) or fibrinous one.
  - Presence of air may suggest infection.
  - Several collections at same time in different stages of evolution mainly in acute pancreatitis.

Necrosis

- Seen as areas of hypoechogenicity with capsule deformation.
- Time of start cannot be predicted.
- The necrosis after about 4-6 weeks organizes to form pseudocyst in about 2% cases.

Pseudocyst

- Space occupying structure with thick-wall (2 mm) echoes within indicates sequestra from necrosis.
- *Superinfection*: It may be seen as air not a convincing mode.

Vascular Examination

- About 10-15% cases with pancreatic pathology may have portal and/or splenic vein thrombosis.
- In portal vein thrombosis its diameter increases and echoes may be seen recent thrombosis—slight echoes but in old intense echoes are seen.
- Doppler signals may be absent.
- Splenic vein thrombosis is indirectly diagnosed as splenomegaly with exacerbation of color signal in arteries and vein at hilum and in spleen.
- Pseudoaneurysm of gastroduodenal artery seen as hypoechoic area in head of pancreas.

Conclusion

The examination should be performed at regular intervals to evaluate progression of disease and complications and correlate clinically.

BOWEL ULTRASOUND

In ultrasound of bowel we mainly concentrate on visualizing small intestine, mesentery, and colon and added information of lymph nodes and vascular supply by use of Doppler.

Probe

Low frequency curvilinear (3.5-5 MHz) probe used for standard exam of abdominal structures, but in some cases high frequency (7.5-10 MHz) probes, used for abdominal wall exam and superficial collections

What Do We Assess?

- Thickness of bowel wall asymmetrical or symmetrical.
- Motility (peristalsis)
- Transmural changes
- Vascularity mainly mesenteric
- Lymph nodes in vicinity.

Structure and Appearance of Normal Bowel

- Bowel is seen as alternating band of light and dark zones.
- *Serosa*: Hyperechoic seen as fine bright line.
- *Muscularis propria*: Hypoechoic seen as dark band.
- *Submucosa*: Hyperechoic bright line.
- Mucosa is hypoechoic and interface is hyperechoic.
- No Doppler signal is seen in normal bowel.
- Bowel can be shifted and compressed with probe.
- Normal thickness is less than 3 mm. It is measured from mucosal luminal interface to outer edge of mucosa which is hypoechoic.
- Normally bowel contents move forward and there is no gas within lumen.
- However, in large bowel peristalsis is not well appreciated, air within the lumen may give the appearance of clouds.
- Haustra are seen as greyish extension from wall (Fig. 7.9).

Pathological Conditions

- *Air*: In abdomen and bowel is not normal.
- Air in bowel— anterior bowel wall seen as bright stripe followed by artifacts. Posterior wall will not be seen.
- Air in abdominal cavity— free air against the peritoneal lining will enhance the brightness of peritoneal strip and reverberation artifacts can be seen ringing down from peritoneal lining. It indicates bowel or gallbladder perforation.
- One should distinguish between intraperitoneal air and intraluminal air.

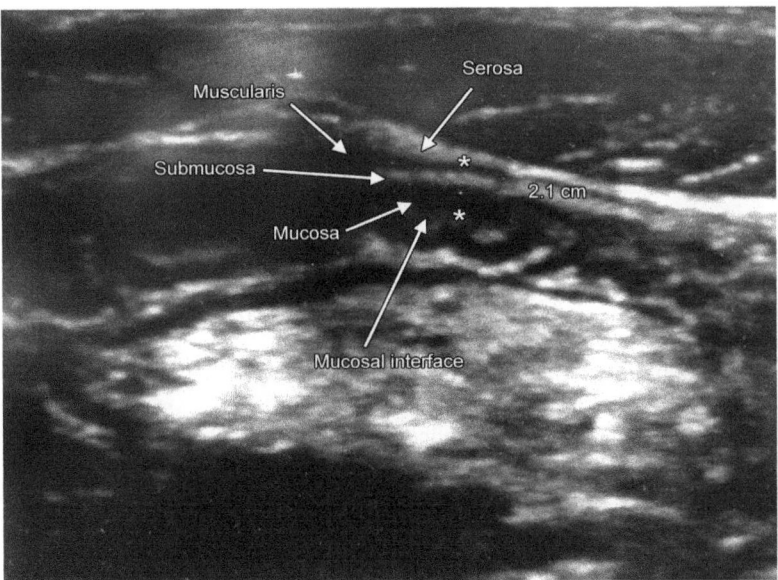

Fig. 7.9: Normal bowel: various layers.

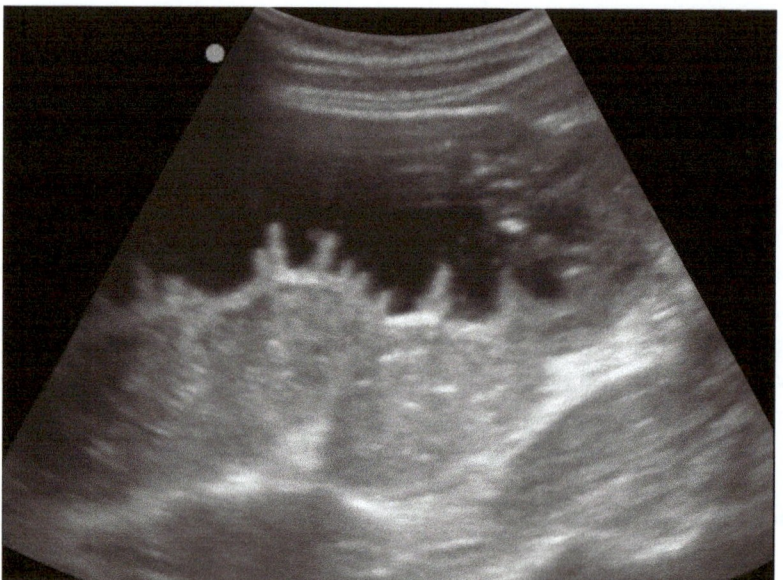

Fig. 7.10: Dilated bowel with contents.

Diverticulitis

Looks like protrusion from colon wall which has ill-defined margins and there is loss of typical bowel wall structure (alternate bright and dark structure).

Bowel Obstruction or Intestinal Obstruction

- The bowel content moves to and fro within the bowel and not as forward propulsion.
- Bowel wall thickening seen as increase in thickness (Fig. 7.10). It may be diffuse segmental or focal circumferential or partial circumferential.
- Seen in tumors, edema hemorrhage, inflammatory condition of bowel.

FURTHER READING

1. Department of ultrasonography, 3rd medical clinic University of medicine and Pharmacy, Cluj-Napoca.
2. Bowra J, McLaughlinc RE. Gallbladder and bile duct. Emergency Ultrasound, pp. 87-97.
3. Romanian Journal of Gastroenterology 2005;(14(1):83-9.
4. Ultrasonography in ICU Practical applications (editor). Paula Ferrada: chapter 5 by Jamie Jones Coleman, pp. 95-109.
5. Radu Badea, USG of acute pancreatitis–Abstract an Essay in images.

CHAPTER 10

Ultrasound in the Neurocritical Care Setting

Pradeep D'Costa, Kedar Toraskar

BACKGROUND

Ultrasonography bedside ultrasound performed by the emergency physician is an extremely important tool that plays a large role in the diagnosis, monitoring and outcome of the neurocritical patients. It is a noninvasive method, is cost effective, is reasonably accurate, and can be easily repeated at bedside. This improves the patient safety, ensures rapid, swift, and correct decisions are taken which can make a difference of life and death in the ICU, emergency room, operating theater or even in the field!

Many a times a patient in altered sensorium poses difficulties in conduction of a detailed neurological examination, these clinical parameters are many times restricted to examination and assessing for brainstem reflexes, cranial nerves, use of scales like Glasgow come scale (GCS), alert, verbal response, pain response, unresponsive (AVPU) scales, many a time near catastrophic events get missed by this approach!

Hence, the clinician relies on presently available tools like CT scan, MRI scans, and invasive intracranial monitors to identify such serious events.

Although of considerable value, the main risks involved in these modalities is related to the transfer of the critically ill patient for the study. Many times these patients are on high ventilatory requirements, high vasopressor supports and hence even slight movements, leave alone transport could lead to a serious emergency, which indeed could compromise the life of the patient! This is in addition to the risk of radiation related exposure for the patient[1,2] and risk of an invasive procedure[3,4] such high risk patients, due to their instability can also cause delays in decision making due to nonimaging due to instability.[5]

Hence we require a more direct, objective, easily repeatable approach, in other words the ultrasound to help us monitor such patients, rapidly, accurately, repeatedly and reproducibly which is the purpose of writing this chapter.

Intracranial blood flows and Doppler imaging of the brain [transcranial Doppler (TCD)], a noninvasive method was started by Aaslid et al.[6] TCD is an invaluable tool in a patient of subarachnoid bleed (vasospasm monitoring), patients of severely raised intracranial pressure (ICP)[7-11] as well,[12] TCD, however, cannot be used as a surrogate for invasive ICP monitor.

Improvement in the quality of machines has now made assessment of the brain parenchyma also possible through the same transcranial acoustic windows.

Even though the clarity of these images is less sharp than the CT/MRI, in an emergency situation, it does give us invaluable information to answer emergency questions about midline shift, fractures, etc.[13-15]

Point-of-care ultrasound in the hands of the intensivist can indeed help us make crucial decisions about raised ICPs, midline shifts, fractures, vasospasms, severe brain injuries/brain death, response to interventions.

The utility of this Point-of-care ultrasound (POCUS), in remote areas, resource scarce areas, areas of combat, low income countries is immense and outcomes are indeed rewarding! The following article presents a brief overview of the spectrum of applications that can be done at the bedside with the ultrasound machine.

VISUALIZATION OF THE ORBIT AND CONTENTS

The full globe and contents can be seen and imaged quite well by the ultrasound.

Basics

- The globe consists of the anterior chamber and posterior chambers.
- The anterior chamber includes the cornea, lens, and supporting structures.
- The posterior chamber is composed of the vitreous humor, retina, and then optic nerve, which will be discussed later.
- Posterior segment is filled with the vitreous humor which is enclosed within the hyaloid membrane.
- Anterior part of the hyaloid membrane is attached to the posterior lens capsule and the posterior part is adherent to the lining membrane of the retina.
- Posterior segment also consists of the retina, choroid, and sclera. Normally all three are adherent
    - The retina extends from the optic nerve till the ora serrata (this is the most anterior part around three-fourths area till iris).
    - The choroid is anchored at the scleral spurs just anterior to the ora serrata and behind close to the optic disk.

Knowledge of these attachments is paramount in our understanding of the various detachments of the eye.

Centrally, we have the optic nerve sheath which passes from the posterior part of the globe to the brain.

Hence, we can identify lens dislocations, abnormalities/foreign bodies in the anterior chamber, vitreous hemorrhage, and retinal detachment by the use of ultrasound in addition to other abnormalities.

Detailed discussions on the same are beyond the purview of this chapter and hence are not discussed.

Only some examples are posted in the Figures 10.1 to 10.4.

Ultrasound in the Neurocritical Care Setting 119

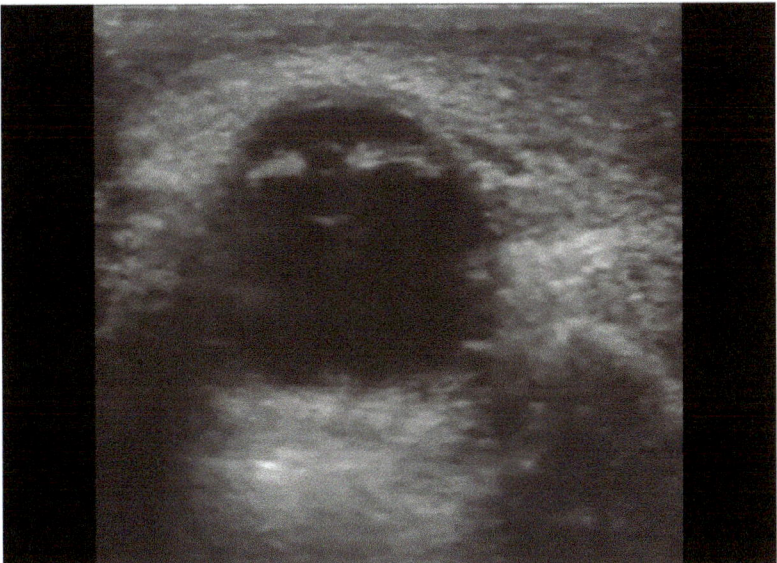

Fig. 10.1: Ultrasound image of the eye/contents.

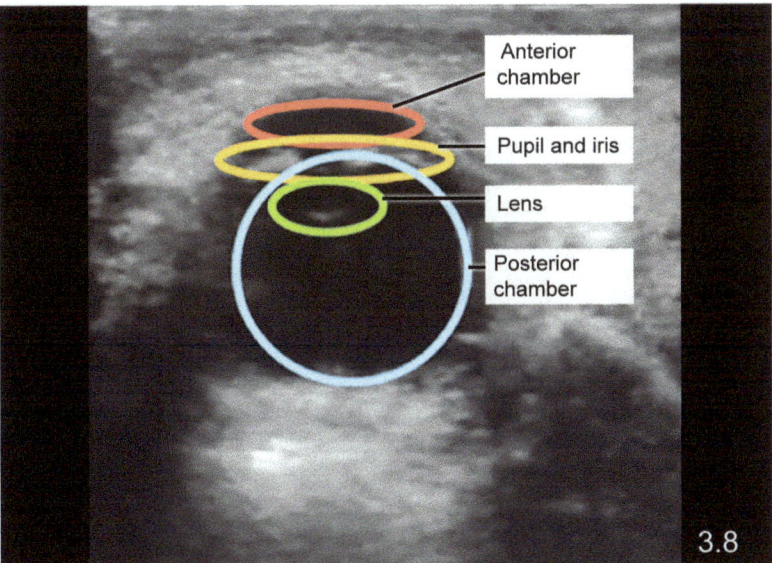

Fig. 10.2: Components of ultrasound of eye area.

Pupils and Reaction

- Sometimes the critically ill patient, due to trauma to the face region, develops swelling of the periorbital tissues.
- This, many a times, creates difficulties in opening the eyes to examine the pupils.

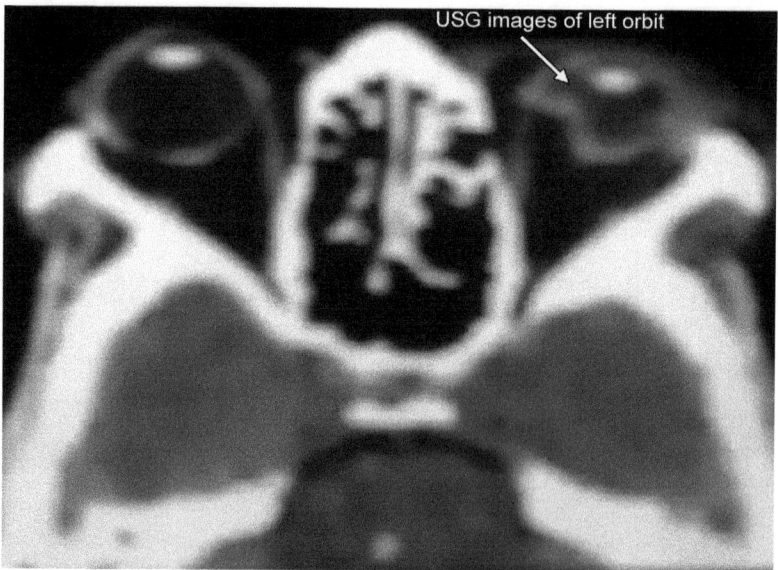

Fig. 10.3: CT scan of left orbital trauma.

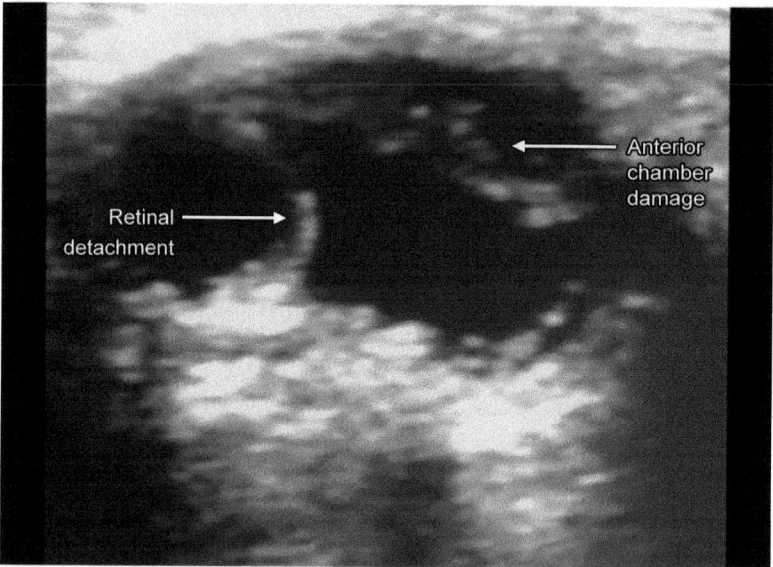

Fig. 10.4: Ultrasound image of left orbital trauma.

- The ultrasound machine can be a very valuable tool in such situations.
- The correct size, shape, and reaction to light can be accurately estimated by the use of the ultrasound (commonly the linear probe is utilized for this application)
- The attached Figures 10.5 and 10.6 elaborate the points.

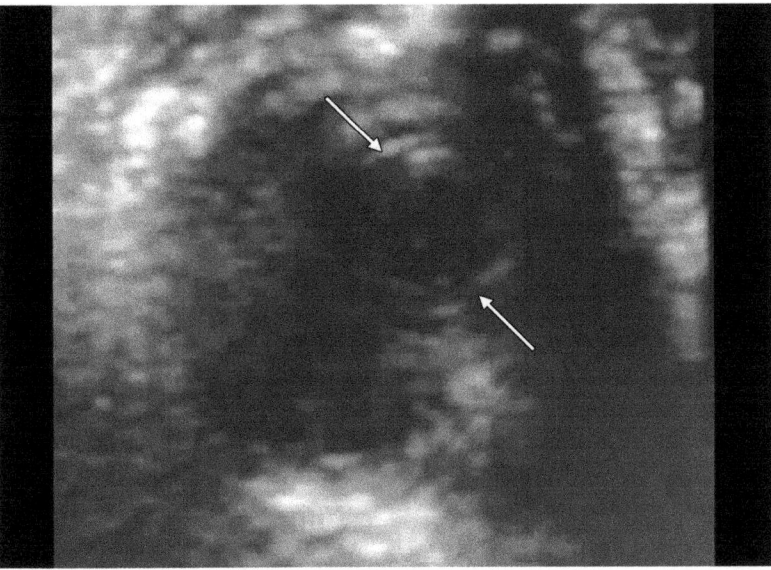

Fig. 10.5: Dilated pupil.

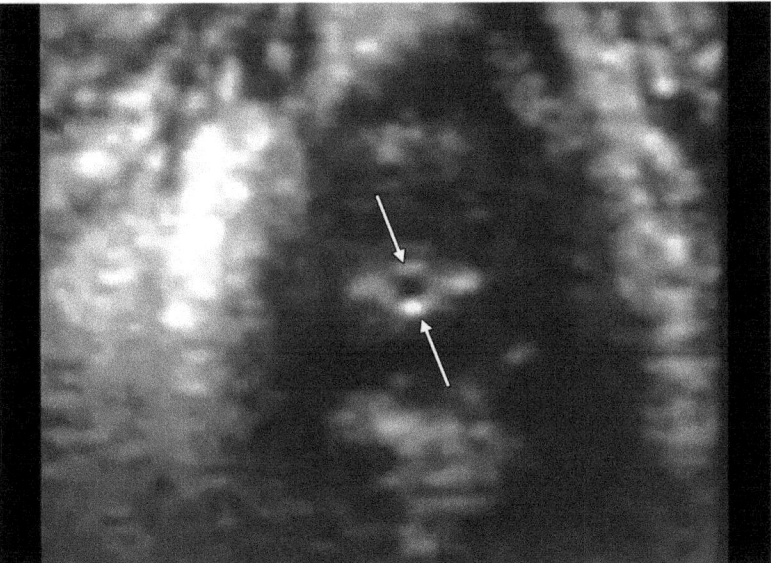

Fig. 10.6: Constricted pupil.

Optic Nerve Sheath

Optic Nerve Sheath Diameter Measurements and the Correlation with Raised Intracranial Pressures

Many recent studies have shown great promise in measuring the optic nerve sheath diameter and correlating it as a surrogate marker (through the orbital view) of raised ICPs. The optic nerve in its most distal portion is covered by the dura, this is known as the optic nerve sheath. It follows that changes in the ICP would have the effect on the intracranial dural space, and then get transmitted to the optic nerve sheath, which indeed is an extension of this dural space. Hence, dilation of the sheath or swelling of this sheath could be an indirect evidence of raised ICPs! These changes are most prominent in the anterior portion of the sheath, just behind the eyeball, this is an area which can be easily approached by ultrasound through the orbits!

Clinical signs sometimes appear late in cases of raised ICPs, which makes it so much more important to detect these changes early (by ultrasound) and hence act early, and this may translate into better clinical outcomes![16,17]

How to measure the optic nerve sheath?
We usually use a high-frequency linear transducer for the examination.[18] The depth settings are usually adjusted to optimal levels (usually 5-6 cm depth).

After strict aseptic precautions are taken, for the probe and patient (may cover probe with protective sheath, or cover the eye with nontoxic transparent film ("Tegaderm", a commonly used material), we position the probe over the closed eye. Ultrasound gel may be used to improve visualization of the structures. The hypoechoic sinusoid structure running behind the eyeball in a snake like manner is identified as the optic nerve.

For measurement purposes, the cursor is used to measure a point directly perpendicular to the attachment of the optic nerve disk, this line is 3 mm long.

Another line is now drawn perpendicular to this line, which runs from the outer to outer border of the sheath. Care must be taken not to measure the optic nerve diameter, but the optic nerve sheath diameter! This point usually marks the area where pressure changes from the brain is best measured! (Figs. 10.7 and 10.8).[19,20]

Varying reports exist on the cutoff diameter for raised ICPs, some studies mention 5 mm is the cutoff point, and some studies recommend 5-6 mm as a gray zone and 6 mm as a better guide to raised pressures.[16]

In our clinical experience, diameters more than 6-7 mm could suggest raised ICP.

Some indirect measures of raised ICP could be seen with a bulging fundic papilla or bulging optic nerve sheath.

Recent literature describes excess tortuosity of the optic nerve as a possible sign of raised ICP, but more data is required before conclusions are drawn.

Another sign which has been described in literature is the "crescent" or "doughnut" sign.

Calculations of the optic disk width using the 30 degree test and evidence of fluid around the optic nerve has been found to be useful in confirming papilledema.

Another interesting study compared the measurement of the optic nerve sheath diameter with the eyeball transverse diameter.

Values of more than 0.19 may be a better indicator of intracranial hypertension and have been studied in cases if intracranial bleeds than optic nerve sheath diameters alone.[21]

VISUALIZATION OF THE SINUSES

Many a times, patients in the critical care unit have troublesome pyrexial diseases which are difficult to diagnose.

One important cause of such a febrile illness which many times goes unexplored is sinusitis.

Ultrasound in the Neurocritical Care Setting 123

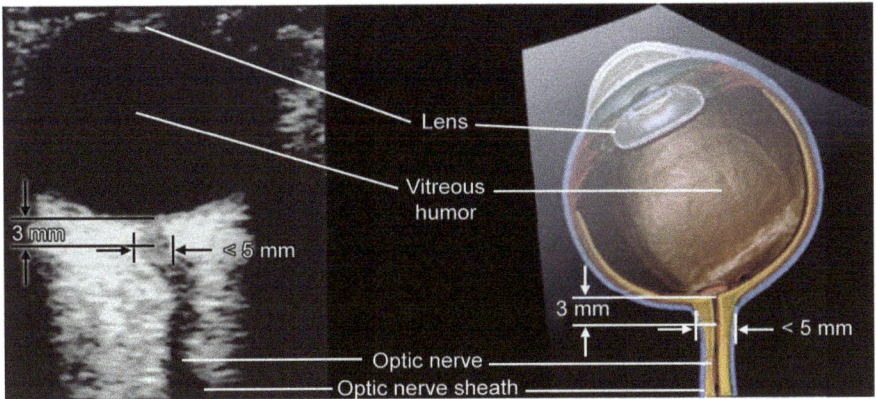

Fig. 10.7: Measurement of optic nerve sheath diameter.

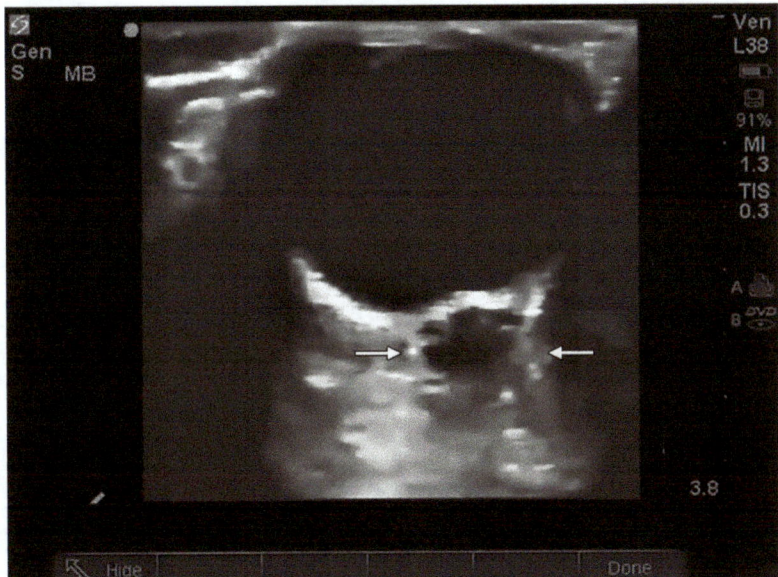

Fig. 10.8: Raised intracranial pressure and dilated optic nerve sheath.

Basic

The sinuses are air filled organs, hence visualization of a normally aerated sinus is difficult to visualize.

Once the sinuses start getting infected, they get progressively filled with fluid/secretions making visualization of the sinuses by ultrasound much more easy.

Normal Sinus

Since the normal sinus is filled with air, the ultrasound picture will look like repetitive artifacts (Figs. 10.9 and 10.10).

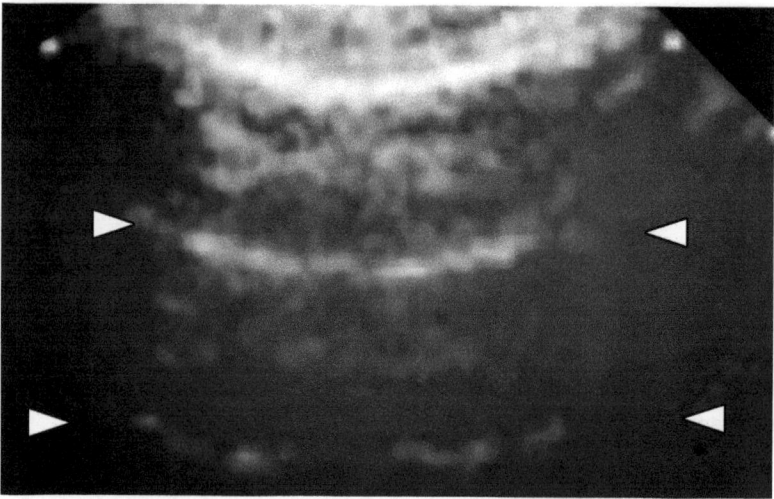

Fig. 10.9: Normal USG appearance of maxillary sinus.

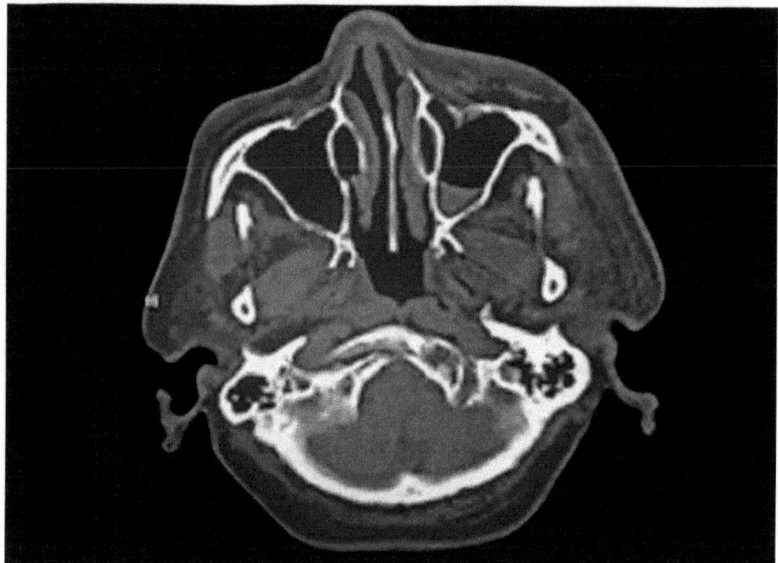

Fig. 10.10: Partial haziness in left maxillary sinus.

Sinusogram

Depending on the fluid/pathology filled sinus, the sinus gets outlined in the ultrasound like a pitcher, when fully filled—the complete sinusogram is seen and when incompletely filled we can see the incomplete sinusogram (Figs. 10.11 and 10.12).

Ultrasound in the Neurocritical Care Setting

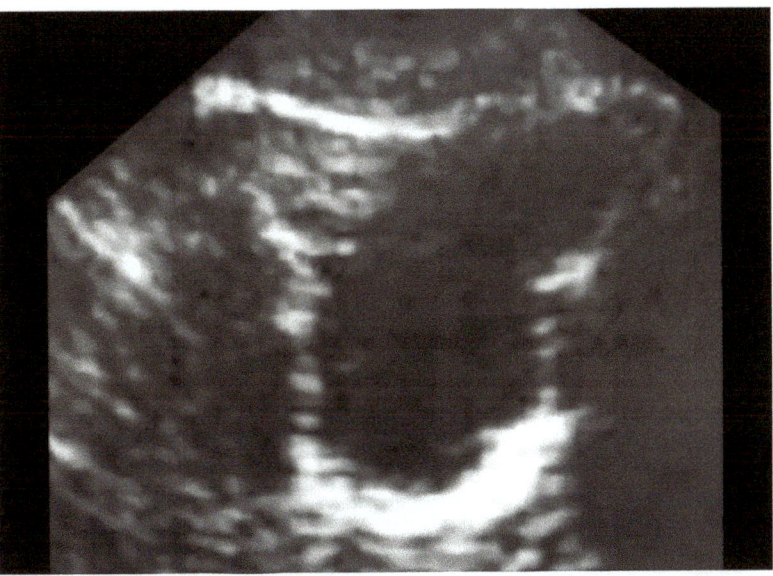

Fig. 10.11: USG image of complete sinusogram.

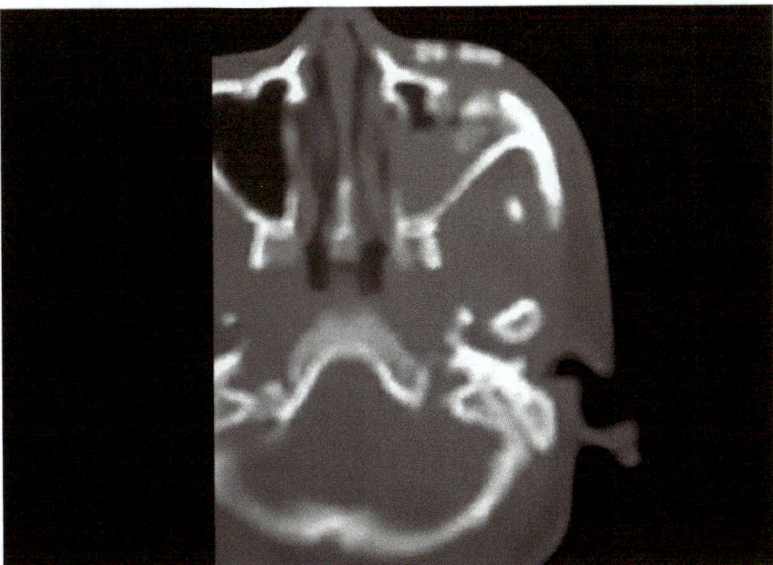

Fig. 10.12: CT scan showing complete left maxillary sinus haziness.

EXTRACRANIAL CEREBROVASCULAR DISEASE (FIGS. 10.13 AND 10.14)

Ultrasound guidance can also be sought for extracranial cerebrovascular disease.

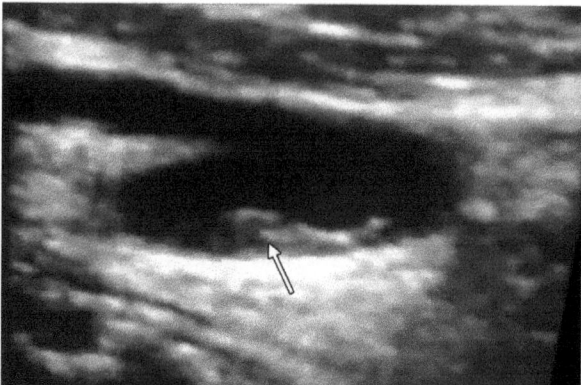

Fig. 10.13: USG image of neck region showing plaque.

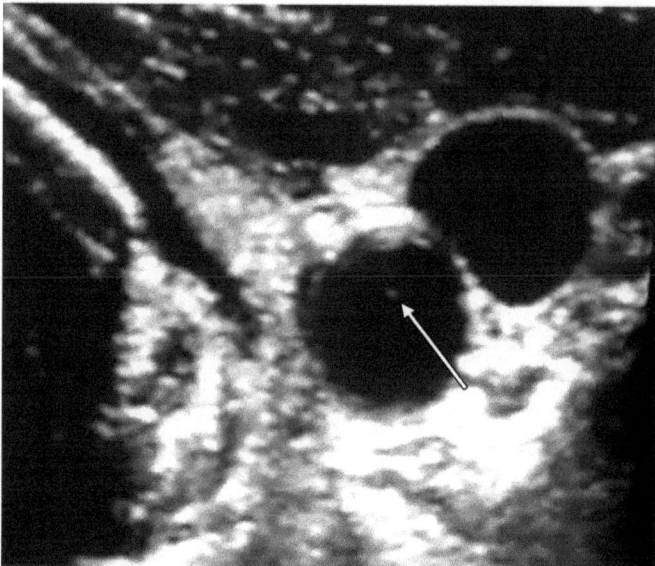

Fig. 10.14: Plaque in carotid artery.

Arteries that can be scanned include the common carotid artery (CCA), internal carotid artery (ICA), external carotid artery (ECA), and also vertebral and subclavian arteries.

Basics

- Mostly, the CCA is medial to the internal jugular vein.
- The CCA bifurcation usually occurs at the angle of the mandible.
- External carotid artery is usually anteromedial to ICA and larger.

- Internal carotid artery and CCA have no extracranial branches, while the ECA has multiple branches.

Identification of the arteries:
- Internal carotid artery—low resistance shallow upstroke and relatively high end-diastolic velocity (EDV).
- External carotid artery—high resistance signal sharp systolic upswing and low EDV.
- Common carotid artery—combination.
- Vertebral—low resistance.
- Bedside assessment of these arteries, many times can provide invaluable clues to the management and decision making in a case of a cerebrovascular accident.
- Just eyeballing and in some cases use of color Doppler signals can identify plaques (which can then be quantified by calcifications, severity, stability, etc.) as well as make a diagnosis of a stenosed artery.
- The same anatomic structures can again be visualized again to see the response to treatment or even to identify if any complications have arisen due to the treatment.
- Expert radiological help can then always be taken to accurately quantify the lesions.

Transcranial Doppler—visualization of the intracranial structures.

Technique

We try to measure the velocity of blood flows within the circle of Willis and vertebrobasilar system through areas of the skull bone which are relatively thinned out in comparison to other areas (commonly temporal area, orbits or foramen magnum).

Spectral analysis of this Doppler frequency is obtained from shifts from the targeted red cells moving through the preselected arterial simple volume area.

Transcranial Doppler then calculates and displays the peak systolic volume (PSV), EDV, and mean volume (MV) on the screen of the studied blood vessel. The pulsatility index (PI) is calculated based on this.

Pulsatility is then described based on the shape of this waveform as normal, abnormal/spiked, and damped.

Pulsatility index values are calculated by inbuilt calculatory mechanisms and interpretations are made:
- 0.8–1.2—normal
- More than 1.2—increased-likely due to raised ICP
- Less than 0.8—reduced—may be seen below a high-grade stenotic lesion are near an AV malformation (supplier)
- Frequency shifts are hence displayed on the Y-axis and time on X-axis.

Basic Anatomy

Internal carotid arteries enter the cranium via foramen lacerum and then branches into anterior cerebral artery (ACA) and the middle cerebral artery (MCA). Both ACA are joined together by the anterior communicating artery (ACOM).

The vertebral arteries of either side join in midline to form the basilar artery. The basilar artery then traverses the ventral part of the pons and ends by dividing into the posterior cerebral arteries (PCAs), right and left. Both the internal carotid arteries are connected to the PCAs by the posterior communicating arteries (PCOM).

This connection then completes the posterior part of the circle of Willis (Figs. 10.15A and 10.16).

Position

Patient must be comfortably resting, supine preferably with head of bed up 30 degrees. However, this examination can be done in almost any position in which the physician is comfortable.

The examiner usually is at the head of the bed, and the patient faces forward.

Views

Commonly used views to insonate the intracranial vessels include:
- Transtemporal (most common and most easy, also gives most wide coverage of the blood vessels)
- Transorbital (restricted, but good in case of nonvisualization of transtemporal route)
- Suboccipital (slightly cumbersome, better to see the posterior circulation)
- Submandibular route (more distal extradural ICA).

Procedure

Choose preselected TCD option on the machine and select the lowest Nyquist level, approximately 20 cm/sec (Fig. 10.15).

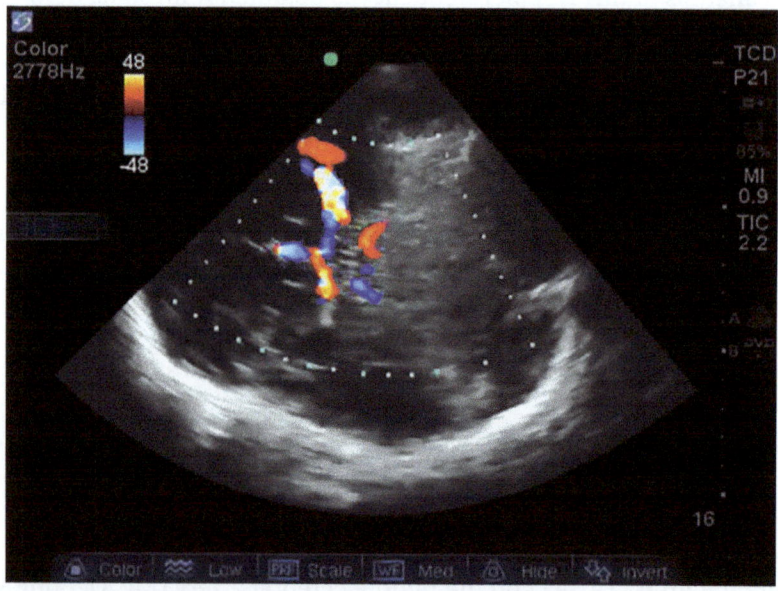

Fig. 10.15: Transcranial Doppler (TCD) showing part of circle of Willis.

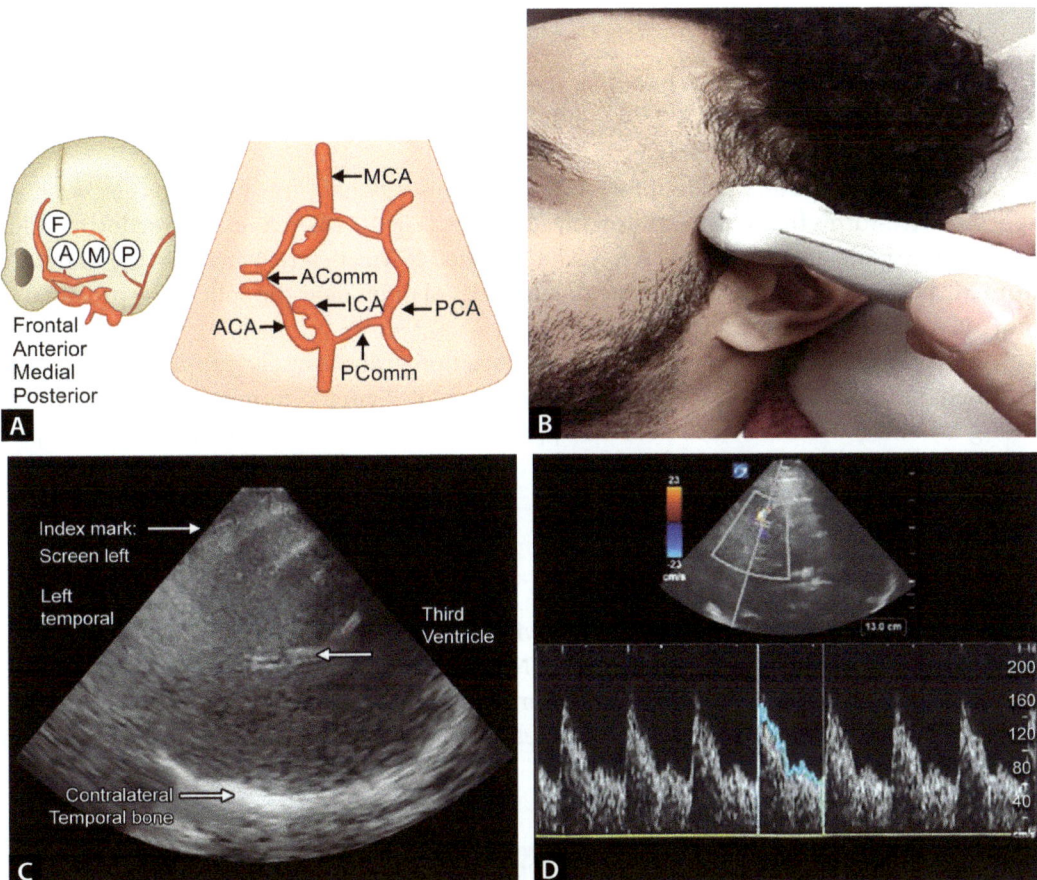

Figs. 10.16A to D: Method for acquisition of transcranial Doppler. (A) Left side shows location of the transtemporal window and its various sections: frontal, anterior, medial, and posterior. Right side illustrates circle of Willis, with middle cerebral artery (MCA) highlighted; (B) Probe index mark orientation toward the patient's anterior/front; (C) Typical 2D image of transcranial Doppler (TCD) from transtemporal window with index mark to screen left, with bright echogenic contralateral temporal bone, and anechoic space of midline third ventricle; and (D) Typical spectral Doppler velocity waveform from MCA, with steep systolic upstroke and step-down diastolic flow (typical mean velocity of 80 cm/s).

For the transtemporal window, place the probe on the temporal aspect of the head, higher to the zygomatic arch, and also above and anterior to the tragus of the ear. There are variations to this approach both horizontally and anteriorly (Fig. 10.16A). Point the marker to the patients anterior surface facing front (Fig. 10.16B). Then orient the marker to the left of the ultrasound screen and locate the temporal bones of both sides (ipsilateral and contralateral). Also locate the third ventricle, which is seen on the images as a midline structure (Fig. 10.16C). Then identify the cerebral peduncles and basal cisterns (appears echogenic).

The MCA now could be located at the top half of the screen, just located laterally to the cerebral peduncle.

(Vessel identification is now based on standard guidelines like cranial window used, depth of sample volume, direction of flow relative to the transducer, relationship of vessel to the junction of MCA/ACA, etc.)

Middle cerebral artery is identified as a red Doppler signal (flow toward), then we obtain spectral wave-forms by using the pulse wave Doppler (Fig. 10.16D). Angle correction should be used. Some guidelines for the MCA location are used to locate it (0.5 cm from M1 and 0.4 cm from M2 parts of MCA. We try to locate the most distal point near the split of the proximal ICA into MCA and ACA, for focal vasospasms intervals.

Angulation of the probe anteriorly from this position (transtemporal) around 6–7 cm should now help us locate the ACA, caudal direction around 6–7 cm the terminal ICA, and posterior tilting around 5–7 cm PCA. Repeat on opposite side to see structures of that hemisphere (Figs. 10.17 to 10.19).

Other views are not discussed here.

Transcranial Doppler Benefits

It is a rapid, radiation free, and noninvasive with minimal transport procedure.

It is reasonably accurate in diagnosis of CNS conditions like vasospasms, stroke (occluded arteries, stenotic lesions, raised ICP, and cerebral circulatory arrest).[13,14] The accuracy too is quite high reaching 89–98% for MCA lesions in the hands of experienced operators accuracy.[13,14]

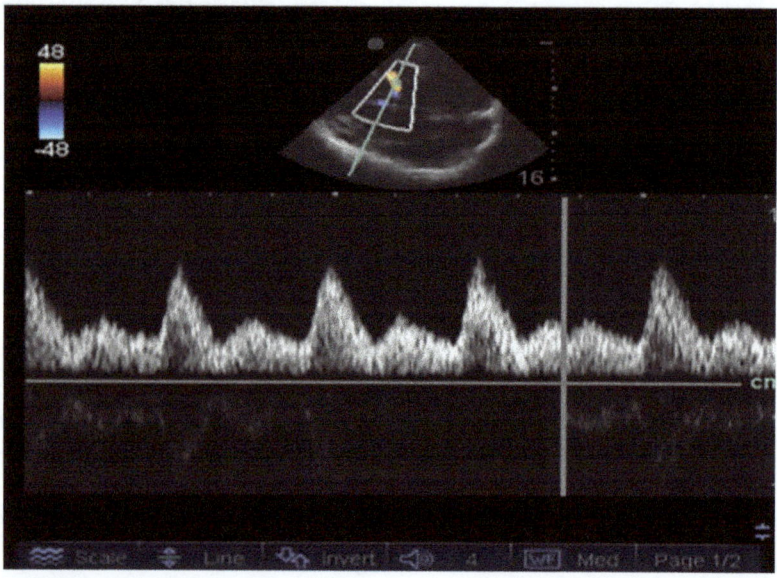

Fig. 10.17: TCD Tracings.

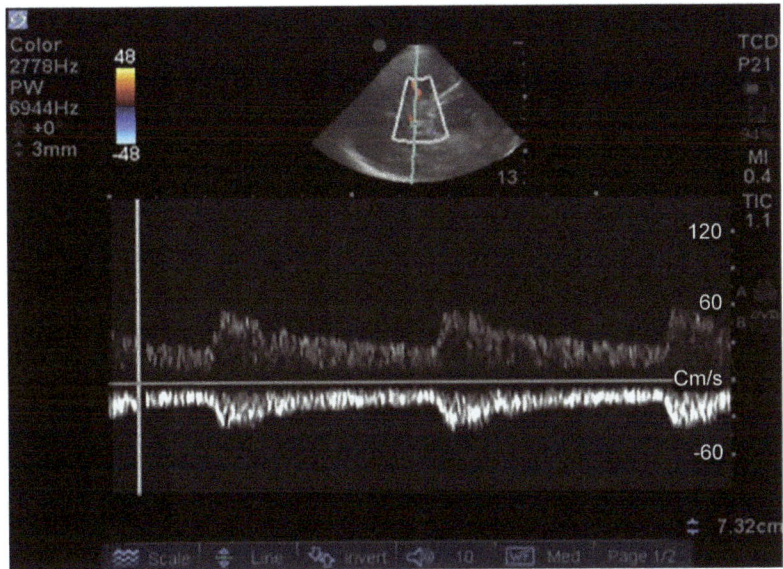

Fig. 10.18: TCD Tracings (bifurcation).

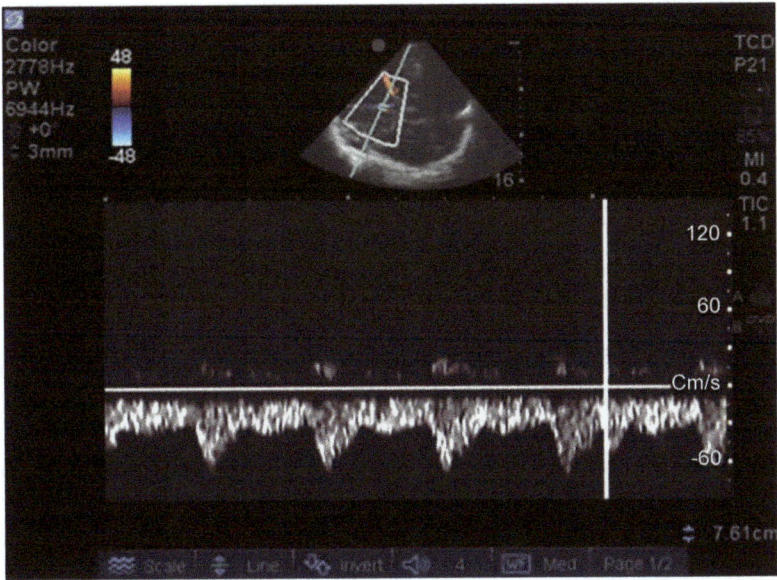

Fig. 10.19: TCD Tracings anterior cerebral artery (ACA).

Midline Shift

Midline shifts can be measured at bedside with the use of ultrasound (studied by Seidel et al.).[15] These measurements correlated reasonably well with the CT scan findings, and are shown to be predictive of a poor outcome in patients of IC bleed, severe brain injuries and strokes.[15,22,23]

Difficulty in visualization of the structures is due to the thick cranial vault and can occur in around 5-20% subjects as per some studies.[13,14]

VASOSPASM DIAGNOSIS AND MONITORING

Transcranial Doppler has been used and studied in great detail in patients who have vasospasm. The clinical scenario, this occurs most commonly in subarachnoid hemorrhage.[6,7,18,24-37] Vasospasm occurs reasonably frequently post-SAH and if not diagnosed early or in time can cause poorer prognosis due to delayed cerebral ischemia and secondary strokes (mortality 15-20%).[8]

Vasospasm is graded as mild, moderate, and severe based on the TCD mean velocities and blood vessel diameter (inversely related).[22,30,33]

The mean velocity of the MCA is less than 80 cm/sec, the normal waveform has a sharp systolic upstroke and a more gradual diastolic deceleration phase.

The vasospasm can be graded as follows:[6,9,25]
- Mild—mean velocities 120-159 cm/s
- Moderate vasospasm 160-199 cm/s
- Severe vasospasm more than 200 cm/s.

Some authors have suggested a change from the baseline mean velocity of more than 21 cm/s per 24 hours during the first 72 hours to be diagnostic of vasospasm.[36]

Vasospasm causing clinical signs is mostly seen is with mean velocities of 160 cm/s.[35]

Vasospasm may also be graded based on the "Lindegaard ratio" formula:[33]
- Lindegaard ratio = Ipsilateral MCA mean velocity/ipsilateral extracranial ICA mean velocity.
- This ratio helps differentiate hyperemia and true vasospasm (hyperemia can be caused by medicines or post interventions
- The following interpretations are possible:
- Lindegaard ratio > 3 = Vasospasm (increase in flow in cerebral blood compared to carotids)
- Lindegaard ratio = 3-5 = Mild-moderate vasospasm
- Lindegaard ratio > 6 = Severe vasospasm.

The MCA is the best in terms of sensitivity and specificity (89-98%) as compared to the CT angiography for the identification of vasospasm, the ACA and PCA are less accurate in mirroring the vasospasm as is also the case with the basilar and vertebral arteries (Fig. 10.20).

All studies mainly done by transtemporal windows.[35,36]

Ideally all the arteries should be interrogated to completely exclude vasospasm.[6]

Intracranial Pressure Estimations

Intracranial pressure, for simplicity, will follow three stages: (1) early, (2) middle, and (3) late.

Each of these changes in the ICP will produce quite characteristic changes in the TCD waveforms (10.21).

Ultrasound in the Neurocritical Care Setting

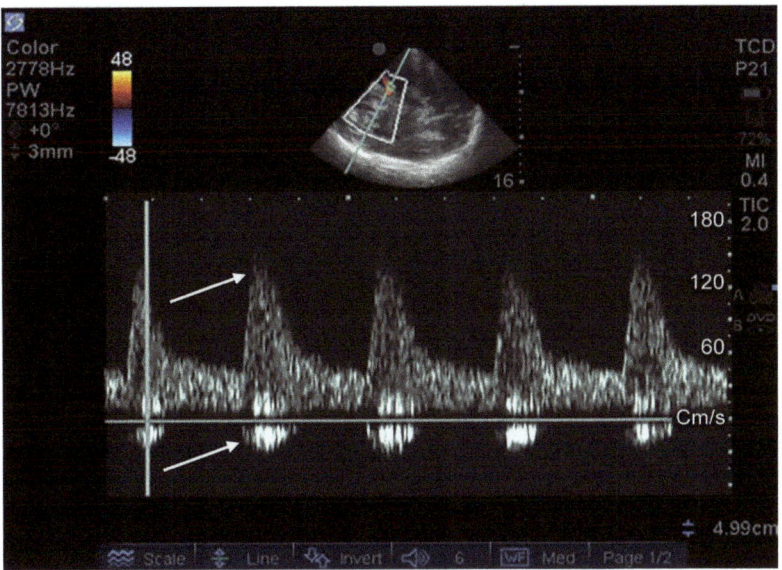

Fig. 10.20: TCD tracing showing raised ICP/diastolic reversal.

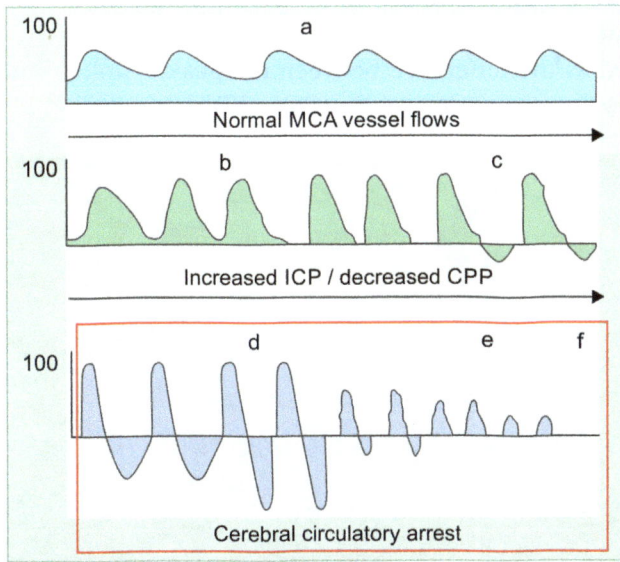

Fig. 10.21: Progression of intracranial circulatory arrest via transcranial Doppler of middle cerebral artery flows [a: Normal systolic upstroke with normal step-down of diastolic flow; b: Increased peak systolic flow with decreasing diastolic flow and eventual blunting of diastolic flow; c: Diastolic flow reversal; d: Biphasic or oscillating flow—where diastolic flow reversal approaches equal size to systolic flow; e: Isolated sharp systolic peak flows of less than 200 ms and small systolic amplitude of less than 50 cm/s; f: Zero flow—where there was previously documented transcranial Doppler (TCD) flow. The red box denotes states (d, e, and f) in which cerebral circulatory arrest can be diagnosed].

Early Stage

Systolic velocities increase and diastolic velocities reduce with increased pulsatility. There is no change in mean velocity.

Middle Stage

As the ICP increases further, the systolic velocities continue to be elevated, but the diastolic velocities start reaching the zero mark due to reduced diastolic flows.

The diastolic pressure of the microcirculation now becomes close to the intracranial tissue pressure.

Late Stage

Reversal of diastolic flows is now seen.

This is due to extremely raised external pressures, exceeding the normal forward flow in diastole, and leading to flow reversal (Figs. 10.22 and 10.23).

GOSLING'S PULSATILITY INDEX

This can be used to estimate the raised ICP.

It reflects the peripheral resistance.

It is calculated as the difference between the peak systolic velocity and end-diastolic velocity divided by the mean velocity [PI = (PSV – EDV)/MV]:[10,34-36]

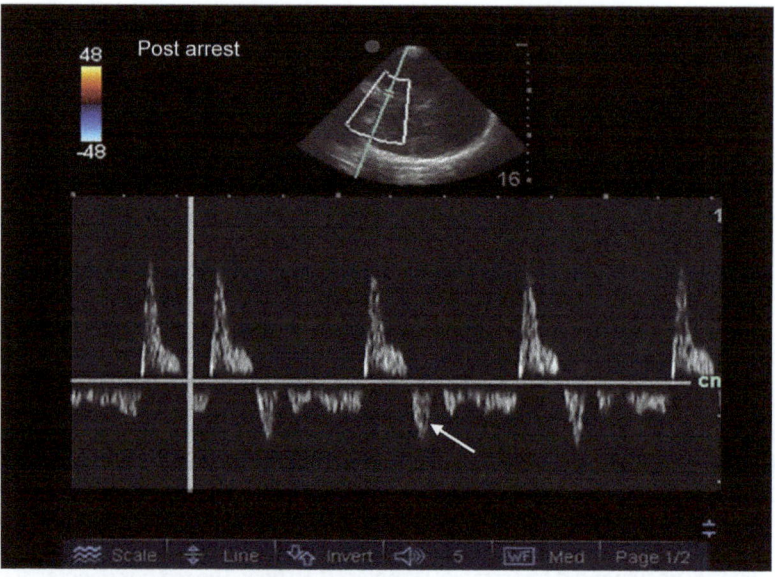

Fig. 10.22: TCD tracings raised ICP and diastolic flow reversal.

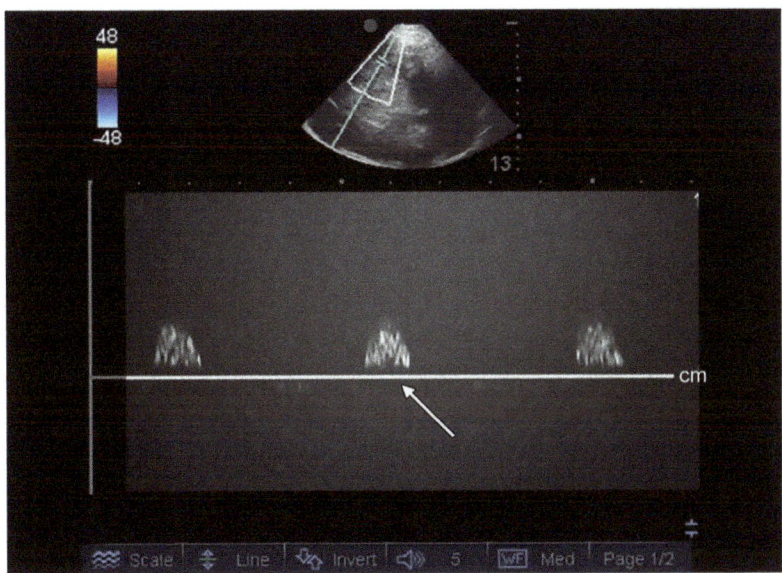

Fig. 10.23: TCD tracings—cerebral circulatory arrest.

Rough estimates of the actual values of ICPs can be obtained by a formula.

The pulsatility index is converted to ICP by this formula (sensitivity and specificity 89%, 92%, respectively).[7]

Pulsatility index > 2.13 = approximate ICP > 22 mm Hg (this is the rough pressure where cerebral perfusion would be getting compromised).[10,38]

Pulsatility index i = < 1.2 = normal = ICP of about 12 mm Hg. The normal ICP measures between 5 mm Hg and 15 mm Hg).[25]

Angulations of interrogating the arteries do not affect the PI, this is a big advantage.[13]

However, the TCD PI has wide range of confidence intervals compared to standard ICP monitors and hence must be carefully interpretated.[13,22,39] The PI can also be affected by changes in arterial carbon dioxide levels and arterial blood pressure changes, these changes are independent of ICPs.

Use in Cerebral Circulatory Arrest/Brain Death

Sharp systolic flows, blunted diastolic flows, diastolic flow reversals, and finally no flow (described earlier also) predict the cerebral circulatory worsening (Figs. 10.22 and 10.23).[7,12] Serial tests are done for more accuracy and also to have baseline comparison scans.[12]

Identification of a stage of cerebral arrest (circulation) can be made by observing at least one of the following criteria, measured at least two times and at least 30 minutes between each reading:[37]

- An oscillating waveform showing near equal systolic flows (forward direction) and reversed diastolic flows.
- Appearance of small pointed systolic peaks, with a low peak systolic velocity (<50 cm/sec) and small duration (<200 ms).
- No flow seen in the intracranial vessels (commonly in a documented previous study with flow present), but flow can be documented in the extracranial vessels.

Other more validated methods like CT, four vessel angiography, MRI angiography can be sought in case of doubts.

Although, in India, TCD is still not accepted as a standard test for severe brain injury, and in the criteria for the diagnosis of brain death, a time will come in the near future when it will be is our firm belief (Fig. 10.23).

An important point to be stressed here is that TCD evaluates for cerebral circulation and its progressive compromise, it does not evaluate brainstem function!

Utility of Point-of-care USG Post-decompressive Craniotomy

A patient who has undergone a decompression craniotomy/craniotomy gives us a good window to visualize the brain parenchyma (Fig. 10.24 and 10.25).

This view in clarity can be compared to the transfontanel view which can be obtained in infants and neonates.[40] The transducer is placed, very gently on the unsupported (by bone) area on the cranium.

Measurements are then taken. Midline shifts, hematoma measurements, compression of ventricles and also sulcal effacement can be quite clearly seen by these views.

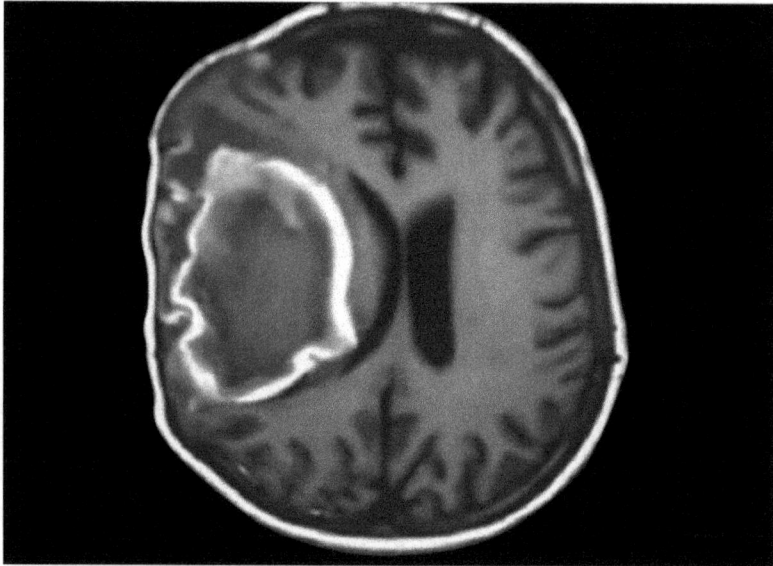

Fig. 10.24: CT scan showing large IC bleed

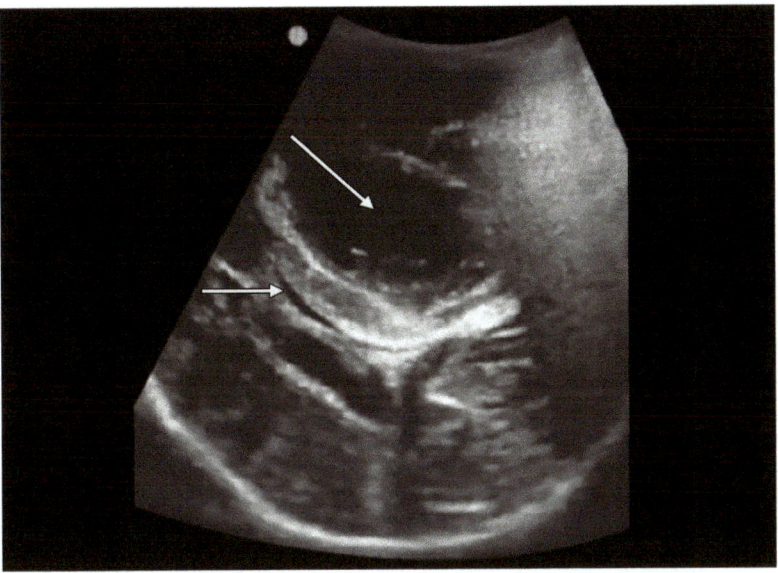

Fig. 10.25: USG image postcraniotomy *(Note:* The compressed ventricles/mass effect)

Again the need for repeated transport of such critical patients can be bypassed for a more safe and of course reasonably accurate method of POCUS.

Catheter placements could also be guided by the use of the ultrasound bedside in such patients.

OTHER USES

Many procedures like lumbar puncture, trauma visualization of cervical/other vertebrae collections within the spinal canal could also be made by ultrasound (some are discussed elsewhere in the book).

CONCLUSIONS

Imaging of the intracranial and some extracranial areas by the intensivist is being increasingly being recognized as an invaluable tool to monitor, treat, and indeed make critical decisions in the neurocritical care unit.

Point-of-care TCD can revolutionize neurocritical care by its varied and simple use. Central nervous system ultrasound performed by non-radiologist specialists is an increasingly available low-cost, versatile and accurate approach that helps improve timeliness and objective decision-making. The advent of non-radiologist performed ultrasound and availability of ultrasound machines now provides a unique climate where point-of-care TCD is a reality. Applications and further uses for the same are being evaluated more and more.

Point-of-care ultrasound is here to stay and revolutionarise our treatment decisions and clinical decision making.

Disclaimer: No conflict of interests.

REFERENCES

1. Andrews PJ, Piper IR, Dearden NM, et al. Secondary insults during intrahospital transport of head-injured patients. Lancet. 1990;335:327-30.
2. Kaups KL, Davis JW, Parks SN. Routinely repeated computed tomography after blunt head trauma: does it benefit patients? J Trauma. 2004;56:475-80.
3. Lieben MA. (2000). Indications for intracranial pressure monitoring. [online] Available from http://online.liebertpub.com/doi/pdf/10.1089/neu.2000.17.479 [Accessed June, 2018].
4. Savers S. Guidelines for cerebral perfusion pressure. J Neurotrauma. 2000;17:507-11.
5. Becker DP, Miller JD, Ward JD, et al. The outcome from severe head injury with early diagnosis and intensive management. J Neurosurg. 1977;47:491-502.
6. Aaslid R, Markwalder TM, Nornes H. Noninvasive transcranial Doppler ultrasound recording of flow velocity in basal cerebral arteries. J Neurosurg. 1982;57(6):769-74.
7. Bellner J, Romner B, Reinstrup P, et al. Transcranial Doppler sonography pulsatility index (PI) reflects intracranial pressure (ICP). Surg Neurol. 2004;62:45-51.
8. Rasulo FA, De Peri E, Lavinio A. Transcranial Doppler ultrasonography in intensive care. Eur J Anaesthesiol. 2008;25:167-73.
9. Rasulo FA, Bertuetti R, Robba C, et al. The accuracy of transcranial Doppler in excluding intracranial hypertension following acute brain injury: a multicenter prospective pilot study. Crit Care. 2017;21(1):44.
10. Cardim D, Robba C, Donnelly J, et al. Prospective study on noninvasive assessment of intracranial pressure in traumatic brain-injured patients: comparison of four methods. J Neurotrauma. 2015;33:792-802.
11. O'Brien NF, Maa T, Reuter-Rice K. Noninvasive screening for intracranial hypertension in children with acute, severe traumatic brain injury. J Neurosurg Pediatr. 2015;16:420-5.
12. Hassler W, Steinmetz H, Pirschel J. Transcranial Doppler study of intracranial circulatory arrest. J Neurosurg. 1989;71:195-201.
13. Moppett IK. Transcranial Doppler ultrasonography in anaesthesia and intensive care. Br J Anaesth. 2004;93:710-24.
14. White H, Venkatesh B. Applications of transcranial Doppler in the ICU: a review. Intensive Care Med. 2006;32:981-94.
15. Seidel G, Gerriets T, Kaps M, et al. Dislocation of the third ventricle due to space-occupying stroke evaluated by transcranial duplex sonography. J Neuroimaging. 1996;6:227-30.
16. Ochoa-Péreza L, Cardozo-Ocampob A. Ultrasound applications in the central nervous system for neuroanaesthesia and neurocritical care. Colomb J Anesthesiol. 2015;43:314-20.
17. Bäuerle J, Lochner P, Kaps M, et al. Intra- and interobserver reliability of sonographic assessment of the optic nerve sheath diameter in healthy adults. J Neuroimaging. 2012;22:42-5.
18. Harrer JU, Eyding J, Ritter M, et al. The potential of neurosonography in neurological emergency and intensive care medicine: monitoring of increased intracranial pressure brain death diagnostics, and cerebral autoregulation—part 2. Ultraschall Med. 2012;33:320-31.
19. Girisgin AS, Kalkan E, Kocak S, et al. The role of optic nerve ultrasonography in the diagnosis of elevated intracranial pressure. Emerg Med J. 2007;24:251-4.

20. Caricato A, Mignani V, Bocci MG, et al. Usefulness of transcranial echography in patients with decompressive craniectomy: a comparison with computed tomography scan. Crit Care Med. 2012;40:1745-52.
21. Qayyum H, Amlakhan S. Can ocular ultrasound predict intracranial hypertension? A pilot diagnostic accuracy evaluation in a UK Emergency Department. Eur J Emerg Med. 2013;20:91-7.
22. Quattrocchi KB, Prasad P, Willits NH, et al. Quantification of midline shift as a predictor of poor outcome following head injury. Surg Neurol. 1991;35:183-8.
23. Motuel J, Biette I, Srairi M, et al. Assessment of brain midline shift using sonography in neurosurgical ICU patients. Crit Care. 2014;18:676.
24. Kiphuth IC, Huttner HB, Struffert T, et al. Sonographic monitoring of ventricle enlargement in posthemorrhagic hydrocephalus. Neurology. 2011;76:858-62.
25. Tsivgoulis G, Alexandrov AV, Sloan MA. Advances in transcranial Doppler ultrasonography. Curr Neurol Neurosci Rep. 2009;9:46-54.
26. Schatlo B, Pluta RM. Clinical applications of transcranial Doppler sonography. Rev Recent Clin Trials. 2007;2(1):49-57.
27. Naqvi J, Yap KH, Ahmad G, et al. Transcranial Doppler ultrasound: a review of the physical principles and major applications in critical care. Int J Vasc Med. 2013;2013:629378.
28. Saqqur M, Zygun D, Demchuk A. Role of transcranial Doppler in neurocritical care. Crit Care Med. 2007;35:S216-23.
29. Topcuoglu MA. Transcranial Doppler ultrasound in neurovascular diseases: diagnostic and therapeutic aspects. J Neurochem. 2012;123:39-51.
30. Van Gijn J, Kerr RS, Rinkel GJ. Subarachnoid haemorrhage. Lancet. 2007;369:306-18.
31. Bleck TP. Rebleeding and vasospasm after SAH: new strategies for improving outcome. J Crit Illn. 1997;12:572-89.
32. Rigamonti A, Ackery A, Baker AJ. Transcranial Doppler monitoring in subarachnoid hemorrhage: a critical tool in critical care. Can J Anaesth. 2008;55:112-23.
33. Lindegaard KF, Nornes H, Bakke SJ, et al. Cerebral vasospasm diagnosis by means of angiography and blood velocity measurements. Acta Neurochir (Wien). 1989;100:12-24.
34. Krejza J, Szydlik P, Liebeskind DS, et al. Age and sex variability and normal reference values for the V(MCA)/V(ICA) index. Am J Neuroradiol. 2005;26:730-5.
35. Mascia L, Fedorko L, terBrugge K, et al. The accuracy of transcranial Doppler to detect vasospasm in patients with aneurysmal subarachnoid hemorrhage. Intensive Care Med. 2003;29:1088-94.
36. Muñoz-Sanchez MA, Murillo-Cabezas F, Egea-Guerrero JJ, et al. Emergency transcranial Doppler ultrasound: predictive value for the development of symptomatic vasospasm in spontaneous subarachnoid hemorrhage in patients in good neurological condition. Med Intensiva. 2012;36:611-18.
37. Lau VI, Arntfield RT. Point-of-care transcranial Doppler by intensivists. Crit Ultrasound J. 2017;9:21.
38. White H, Venkatesh B. Applications of transcranial Doppler in the ICU: a review. Intensive Care Med. 2006;32:981-94.
39. Mayo PH, Beaulieu Y, Doelken P, et al. American College of Chest Physicians/La Societe de Reanimation de Langue Francaise statement on competence in critical care ultrasonography. Chest J. 2009;135:1050-60.
40. Dubourg J, Javouhey E, Geeraerts T, et al. Ultrasonography of optic nerve sheath diameter for detection of raised intracranial pressure: a systematic review and meta-analysis. Intensive Care Med. 2011;37:1059-68.

CHAPTER 11

Ultrasound in Trauma (FAST/eFAST in Trauma Victim)

Pratibha Patel

INTRODUCTION

Point-of-care ultrasound has rapidly changed the outlook for assessment of trauma in emergency and critical care units.

Trauma victims may at times present on admission with distracting injuries, and life-threatening injuries may be present without any warning signs. These injuries may be grave enough and at times need priority and immediate attention for management. This is where role of ultrasound is beneficial.

Physicians have started using this modality since 1970 to aid in various clinical conditions. And gradually ultrasonography (USG) has become initial imaging of choice for trauma care globally and now it has become integral part of "advanced trauma life support (ATLS)".

There are other modalities like roentgenogram and computerized scan. They have certain disadvantages as compared.

Roentgenograms
- Exposure to radiation
- Availability.

CT Scan
- Lack of portability. Needs patient to be shifted
- Expensive
- Exposure to radiation.

WHY USE ULTRASOUND?
- It is easy to learn and perform
- Portable
- Noninvasive
- It does not interfere with ongoing resuscitation
- Rapid and can be repeated as and when required.

Evidence proves that:
Quality improves after 20–25 scans.
- Training includes:
    - Theoretical
    - Practical
    - Supervised scans initially.

It can be used in:
- Prehospital settings
- Disaster management
- During patient retrieval in ambulance, etc.
- Hospital settings
- Emergency department
- Critical care units
- Operation theaters
- Wards.

It can be used by:
- Intensivists
- Emergency physicians
- Trauma surgeons
- Anesthetists
- Radiologists and sonologists.

Ultrasound is used to:
- Assist in identifying blunt and penetrating injuries
- In detecting life-threatening injuries and thus help in directing and prioritizing interventions
- Guiding resuscitations
- Guide interventional procedures ranging from vascular access, nerve blocks to removal of foreign bodies
- In *regional trauma* also USG can give diagnostic information about vast range of pathologies including—individual organs, musculoskeletal, soft tissue and vascular injuries.

The main aim of USG in focused assessment with sonography in trauma (FAST) is to locate free fluid in abdomen and thorax. Specific site of bleeding is of secondary importance.

CURRENT ROLE

In ATLS protocol, FAST examination has to be performed immediately after primary survey. It should not interfere with or delay resuscitation and other treatment.

Role of Ultrasound in Primary Survey

- A = *Airway*:
    - Determine position of trachea
    - Confirm endotracheal tube placement

- B = *Breathing*: Assess for pneumothorax/hemothorax
- C = *Circulation*:
  - Assess for hemoperitoneum
  - Assess for hemopericardium
  - Access for hemothorax
  - To guide peripheral and central venous access
  - Access intravascular filling
- D = *Dysfunction*: Assess optic nerve sheath diameter as a reflection of intracranial pressure
- E = *Exposure*.

FOCUSED ASSESSMENT WITH SONOGRAPHY IN TRAUMA/EXTENDED FOCUSED ASSESSMENT WITH SONOGRAPHY IN TRAUMA

Ultrasound in trauma is now synonymous with FAST/eFAST.

Focused Assessment with Sonography in Trauma

- Term was coined by Rozycki et al. in 1995
- It is a (four viewed) assessment of abdomen
- FAST helps to detect blunt and penetrating injuries of abdomen—hemoperitoneum and hemopericardium.

Extended Focused Assessment with Sonography in Trauma (eFAST)

- Efast detects injuries in thorax—hemothorax and pneumothorax
- A positive fast with high specificity indicates an intra-abdominal injury
- A negative fast (absence of free fluid)—moderate sensitivity does not exclude significant injury.
- At this stage, however, there is little conclusive evidence that its use improves patient survival.

But,
- FAST alters management of trauma patient in following way:
  - Rapid decisions for operative intervention
  - *If negative:* It guides to search for other causes of hypotension
  - It reduces the number of repetitive scans and diagnostic peritoneal lavage (DPL)
  - Probably associated with shorter hospitalization, less complications and lower charges (no studied evidence).

Indication of FAST in Specific Conditions

Blunt Abdominal Trauma

FAST-associated algorithm (Flowchart 11.1): It helps in detecting intraperitoneal bleeding due to trauma to various intra-abdominal organs. The amount of fluid is not important (however

Flowchart 11.1: FAST-associated algorithm. All patients suffering blunt abdominal trauma have a FAST scan and further investigation and management then depends on their hemodynamic status and results of investigations.

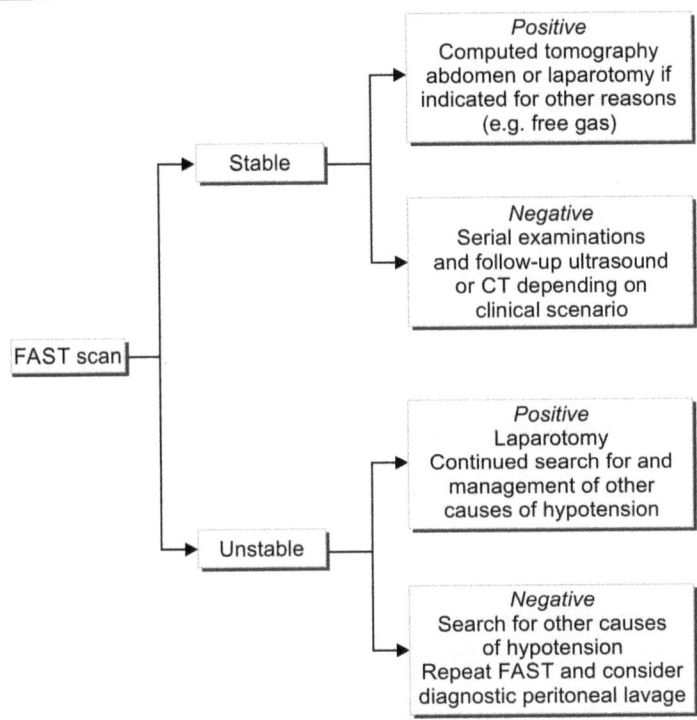

many scores have been put forward), but presence of fluid accounts for injury. In hypotensive trauma patient, FAST screening helps to determine whether bleeding correlates or justifies hypotension. Negative FAST prompts search for other causes of hypotension.
- *Sensitivity*: 90%
- *Specificity*: 99%.

Penetrating Abdominal Trauma

Many studies limit the analysis of abdominal trauma to setting of blunt trauma. However, it is equally useful and negative FAST prompts to look for other causes of hypotension.
- Amount of fluid to be detected and quantification of fluid
- Sensitivity of detecting fluid is volume dependent. Volume required to detect is around 200–300 mL.
- Various scoring systems are there but not yet validated, but can mainly be used as guide for management and surgical intervention.

Huang et al: Amount of fluid expected to be detected around 1,000 mL
- Total 8 points:
  - 1 point for each quadrant—(four quadrants)
  - 2 points—if fluid is more than 2 mm in depth [right upper quadrant (RUQ)/left upper quadrant LUQ]
  - 2 points for floating bowels
  - *Score more than* 3: 96% required surgical intervention
  - *Score less than* 3: 38% required surgical intervention.

Mckenney et al: System based on examination of five areas:
1. Right subphrenic
2. Right subhepatic
3. Left subphrenic
4. Perisplenic
5. Pelvis.

Deepest pocket is measured in centimeters and fluid in other pockets is added as 1 in each pocket.
- *Score more than* 3: 85% require surgery
- *Score less than* 3: 15% require surgery.

Sirlin et al: Fluid in each anatomic region 1 point
- Score more than 3: 63% require surgery
- Score less than 3: 40% require surgery.

Sensitivity 50%:
- *CT scan:* It is better in showing parenchymal injury
- It can differentiate solid organ injury from bowel injury
- Superior in demonstrating retroperitoneal bleeding
- But our aim with USG is to visualize bleeding is present or not.

CARDIAC TRAUMA

Blunt Trauma

- Uncommon.
- Blunt trauma may cause rupture of cardiac structures which leads to instantaneous death. FAST should be performed to rule out pericardial collection.

Penetrating Trauma

All patients with penetrating chest injuries should be screened for cardiac trauma. Development of collection and tamponade may take time as pericardium seals the injury initially, so repetitively ultrasound should be done.
- Sensitivity 100%
- Specificity 97%.

CHEST TRAUMA

Same for both blunt and penetrating trauma.

Hemothorax

- Free fluid accumulation dependent spaces that is costophrenic angle and may displace lung tissue if more
- It can detect around as less as 20 mL of fluid (X-ray requires around 200 mL of fluid) hence more sensitive
- Time taken is less guides chest tube placement
- Fractured ribs can also be seen.

PROBE AND SCAN

- Curvilinear abdominal probe (2-5 Hz) frequency—it has deeper penetration however resolution is less. The curved surface provides better lateral resolution. All views can be seen with this probe.
- But linear probe for viewing pleural space and cardiac (sector) probe for cardiac view are ideal.
- Depth 15-20 cm for hemothorax, hemoperitoneum, hemopericardium, and 5 cm for pneumothorax.
- Adjust the gain so as liver tissue is seen as gray mottled and diaphragm is seen bright translucent.

Ultrasound Windows for FAST (Fig. 11.1)

- Right upper quadrant (RUQ)
- Left upper quadrant (LUQ)
- Pelvic
- Subcostal.

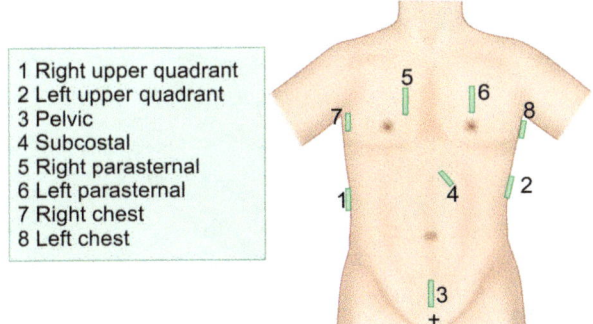

Fig. 11.1: FAST and eFAST views.

RIGHT UPPER QUADRANT VIEW (MORISON'S POUCH OR RIGHT FLANK VIEW)

This view uses liver as an acoustic window. Probe is placed longitudinally where costal margins meet anterior axillary line (8th–11th intercostal space) with marker dot pointing cephalad (head) (Figs. 11.2A and C).

This gives the coronal view of following structures:
- Lower part of lung
- Diaphragm (bright)
- Liver (gray)
- Right kidney
- Hepatorenal space (Morison's pouch) (Fig. 11.2B).

Follow the lower edge of liver caudally till a good view of tip of kidney is obtained free fluid is usually seen in Morison's pouch or lower edge of liver and sometimes above liver, i.e. space between liver and diaphragm.

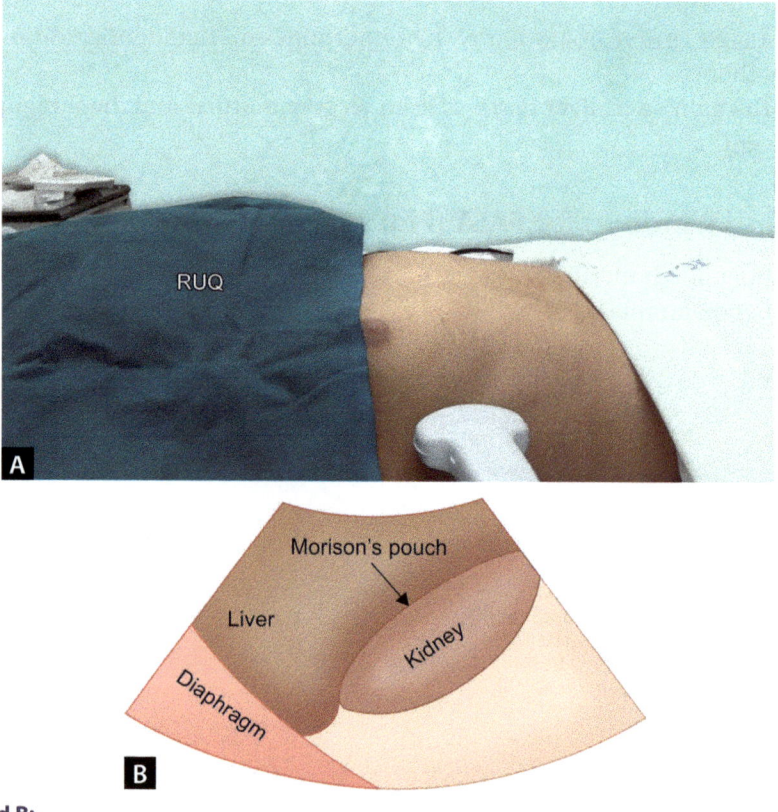

Figs. 11.2A and B:

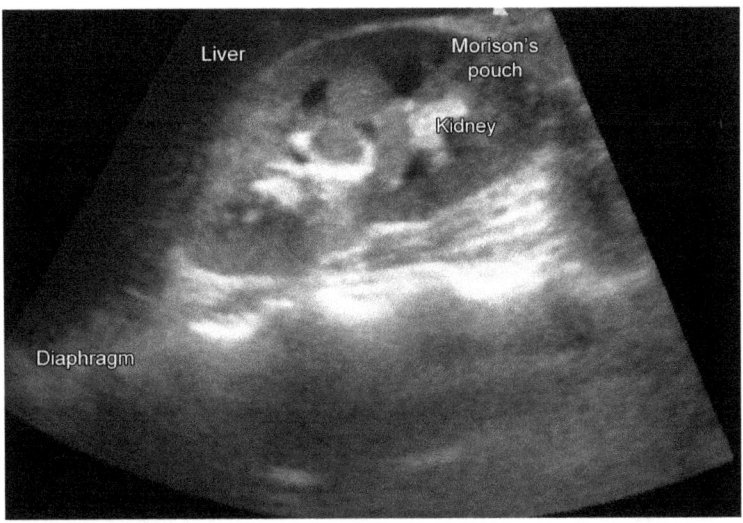

Fig. 11.2C:

Figs. 11.2A to C: Right upper quadrant (RUQ).

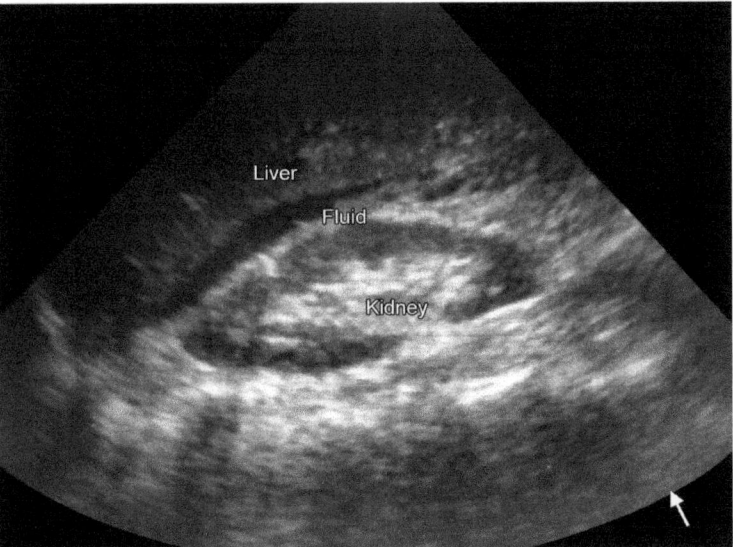

Fig. 11.3: RUQ view showing free-fluid.

Free-fluid will be seen as Black Anechoic Strip (Fig. 11.3)

Diaphragm seen as bright hyperechoic line helps to differentiate between pleural space and peritoneal cavity and also we can appreciate diaphragmatic movement.

The rib shadows may be prominent and obscure the view, this can be minimized by rotating the probe slightly counterclockwise (marker dot pointing toward posterior axillary line).

Free fluid seen only at tip of liver is falsely positive.

Slide the probe cephalad to obtain better view of diaphragm. Pleural fluid if present will be seen as black triangle above the diaphragm and this may also show free intraperitoneal fluid superior to liver.

Caudal movement of the probe will show inferior pole of kidney as well as right paracolic gutter for fluid assessment.

Left Upper Quadrant (Perisplenic or Left Flank View) (Figs. 11.4 and 11.5)

This view uses spleen as an acoustic window.

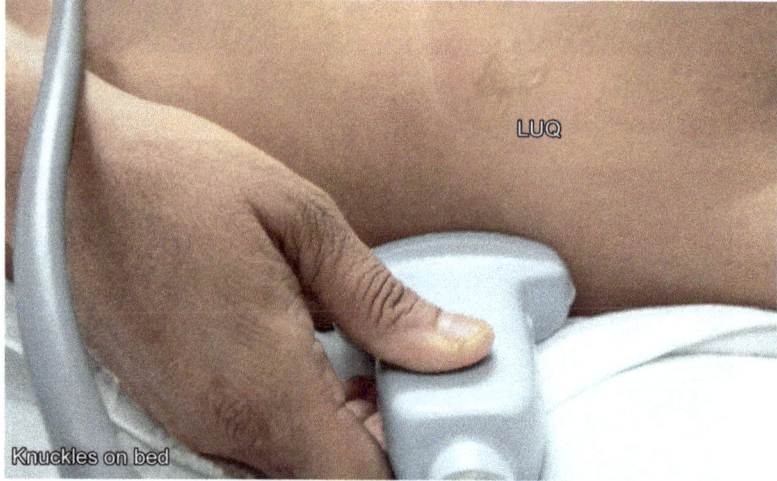

Fig. 11.4: Left upper quadrant (perisplenic or left flank view) (LUQ: Left upper quadrant).

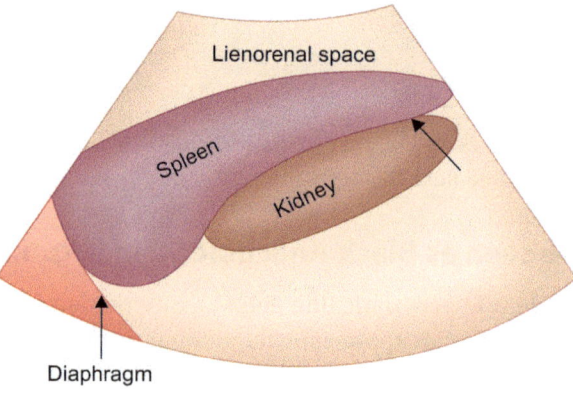

Fig. 11.5: Left upper quadrant.

Probe is placed longitudinally in left side at about 6th to 9th intercostal space (a bit above as left kidney is placed higher as compared to right one) along posterior axillary line with marker dot pointing cephalad (toward head).

This window gives us good coronal view of:
- Spleen
- Left kidney
- Left pleural space
- Space between spleen and left kidney (lienorenal space)
- Diaphragm is a bit difficult to see.

Ribs may sometimes obscure this view, so to get a better view rotate the probe slightly clockwise so that the marker dot points toward posterior axilla ….if still cannot see spleen ask patient to take deep breathe (if conscious).

If free fluid is present, it is more commonly seen surrounding spleen or the space between diaphragm and spleen.

It is uncommon to see fluid in space between spleen and left kidney, i.e. lienorenal space (Fig. 11.6 to 11.8).

Collection between spleen and diaphragm is seen more as this is the most dependent part of the left side of the abdomen.

Pelvic View (Retrovesical Pouch/Retrouterine Pouch or Pouch of Douglas)

It is not as easy to obtain like previous views.

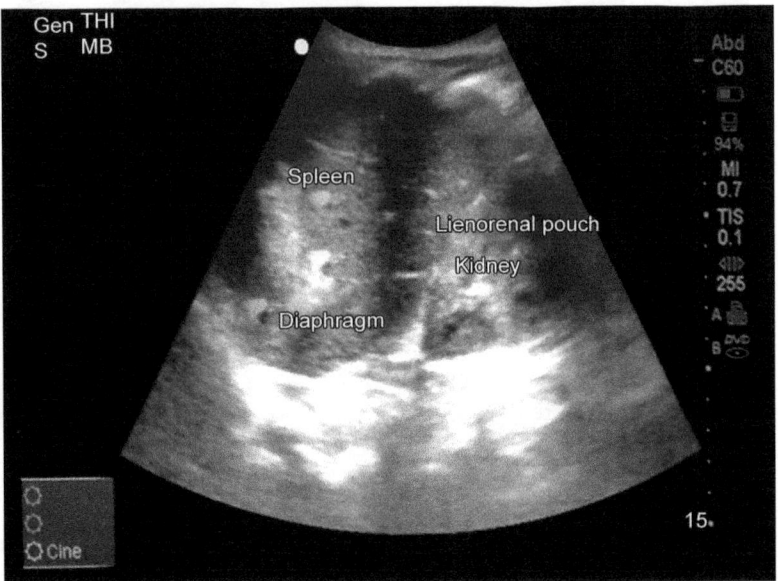

Fig. 11.6: LUQ view with free fluid.

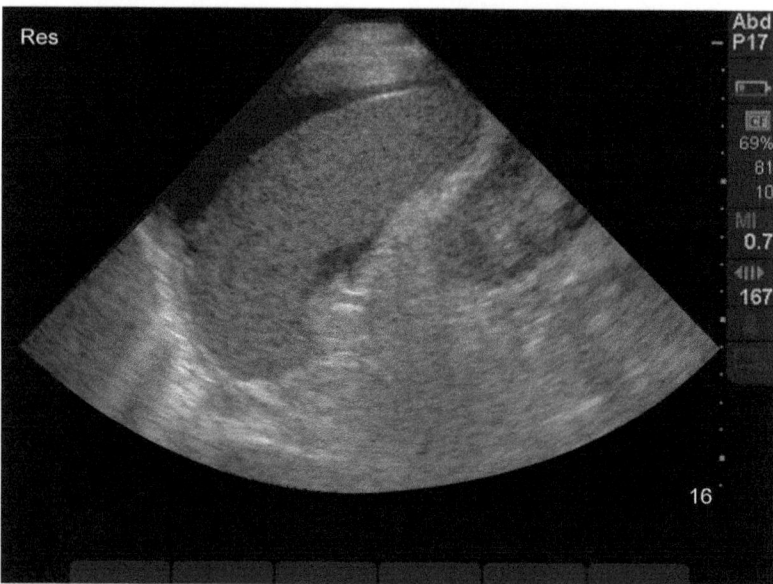

Fig. 11.7: Free-fluid in left upper quadrant.

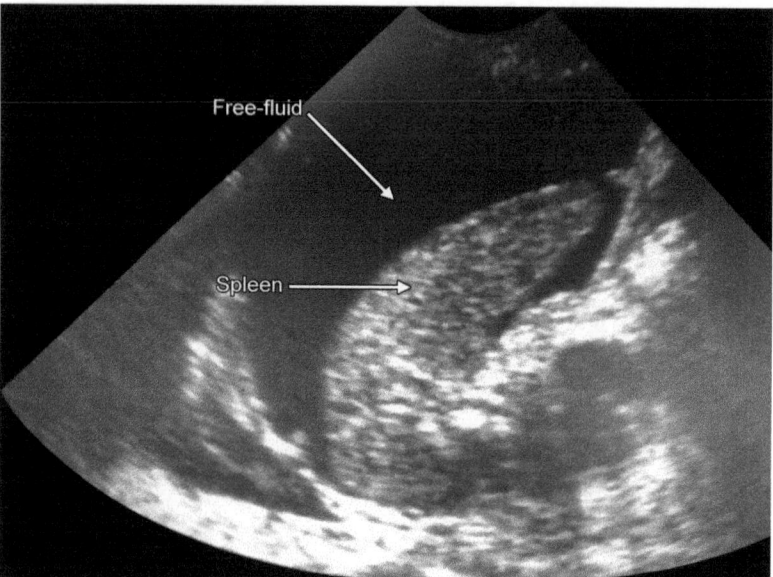

Fig. 11.8: LUQ view free-fluid perisplenic.

It uses urinary bladder as an acoustic window, hence, the bladder must be full or preferably done prior to Foley's catheterization or will have to fill up the bladder with fluid and clamp catheter to get desired view.

Ultrasound in Trauma (FAST/eFAST in Trauma Victim)

Pelvis is the most dependent part in abdominal cavity so fluid tends to get accumulated here. Only bladder is the main structure seen. It can be screened in:
- Longitudinal plane (Fig. 11.9A)
- Transverse plane.

Longitudinal Plane

Probe is placed longitudinally just above pubis symphysis with marker dot pointing cephalad. If not seen properly may have to dip the probe in skin.

Full bladder appears triangular in shape and lower angle of bladder marks the border between the intraperitoneal space and the true pelvic structures.

In males fluid will be seen in between the posterior wall of bladder and peritoneum.

In females, uterus sits just posterior to bladder, hence fluid is seen posterior to uterus (pouch of Douglas).

If bladder is empty, pouch of Douglas may be identifiable but retrovesical pouch is difficult to visualize (Figs. 11.9B and C).

Transverse View

Rotate the probe anticlockwise so that the marker dot points right side of patient. OR probe is placed just above the pubic symphysis with marker dot pointing toward right of patient. Bone is seen as bright structure. From this position slide the probe at 45° caudally so that one can see behind and beyond the bone. If free fluid is present, it is seen posterior to bladder or uterus or adjacent to corners of bladder (Fig. 11.10).

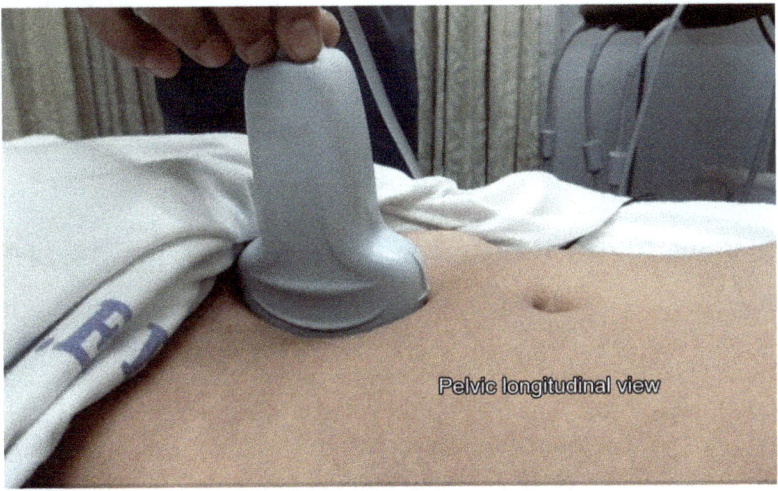

Fig. 11.9A:

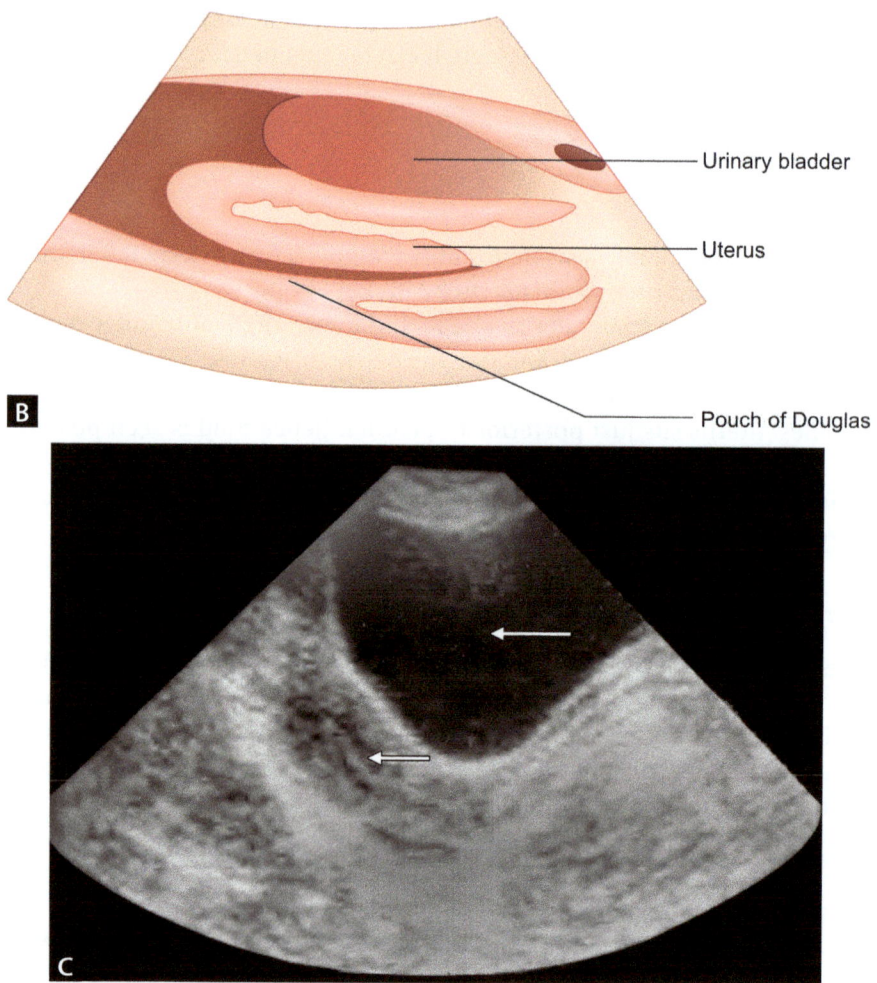

Figs. 11.9B and C:

Figs. 11.9A to C: Pelvic longitudinal view.

Subcostal View: Pericardial or Subxiphoid View (Figs. 11.11A to C)

This uses liver as an acoustic window for cardiac evaluation. In trauma, it is mainly useful to evaluate pericardial cavity and all four cardiac chambers mainly right sided.

It is also used for visualization of inferior vena cava (IVC) and hepatic veins.

Place the probe in subxiphoid region that is just in the notch formed by both side costal margins and lower end of xiphisternum slightly toward right side with marker dot pointing toward left flank that is 3 o'clock position. Dip the probe into the skin so as to get beneath xiphisternum and angle the probe toward left shoulder.

This will give us the view of liver and right ventricle adjacent to each other and right atrium leading to IVC.

Pericardial effusion if present is seen easily as anechoic or hypoechoic stripe between liver and heart or circumferentially around heart.

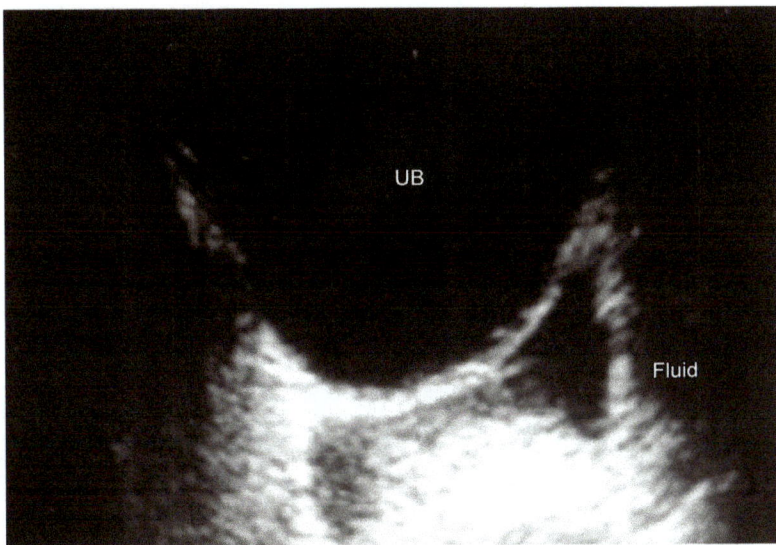

Fig. 11.10: Urinary bladder (UB).

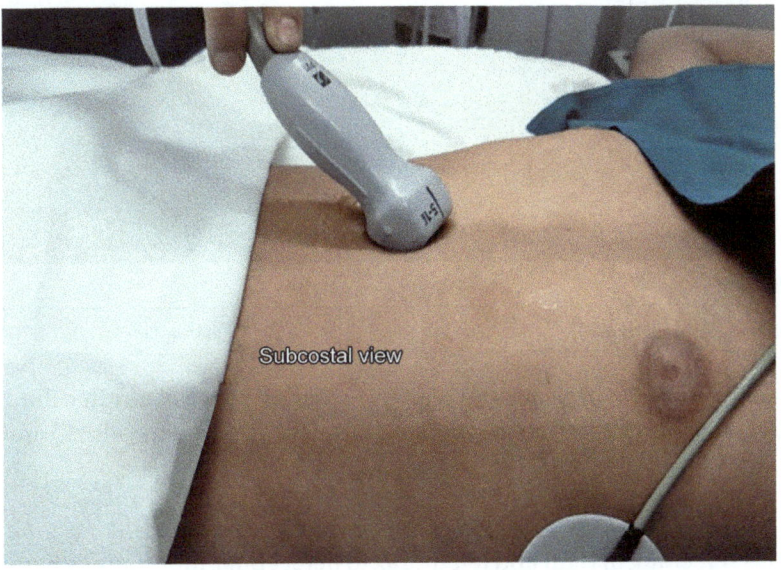

Fig. 11.11A:

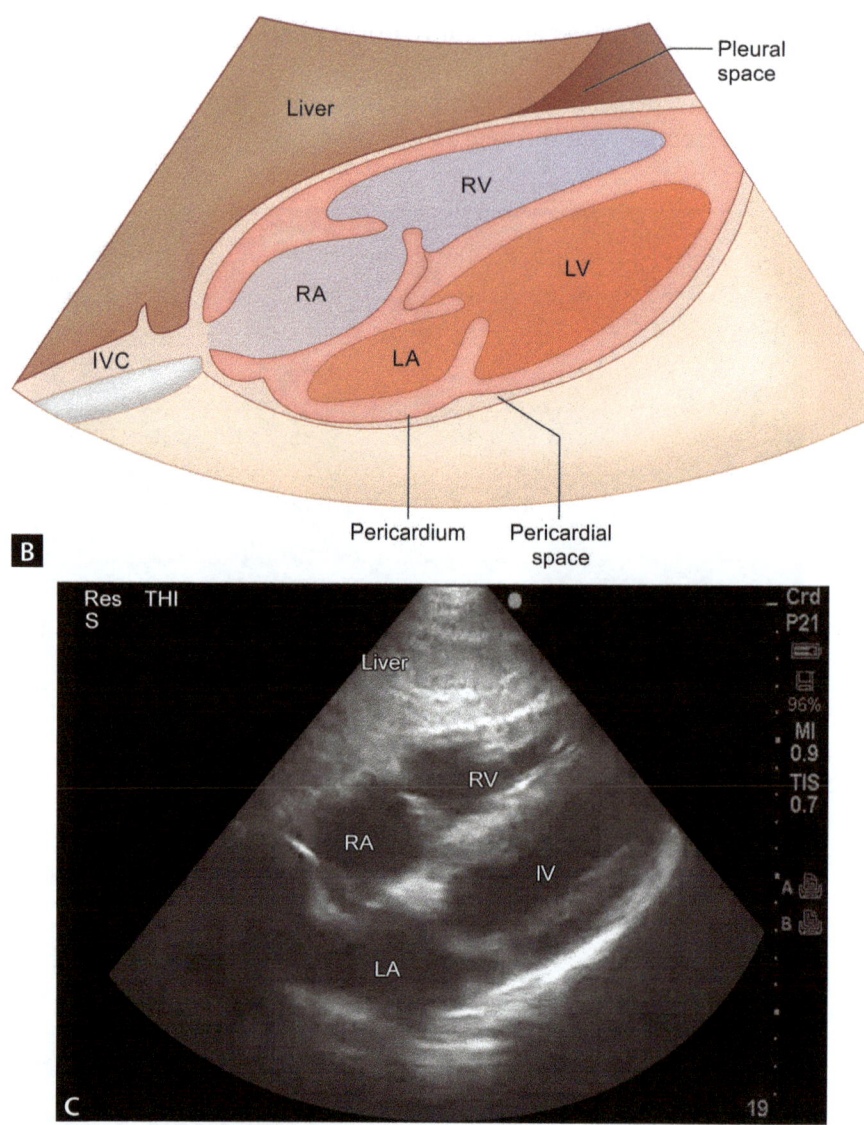

Figs. 11.11B and C:

Figs. 11.11A to C: Subcostal view.

The potential space of pericardium is analyzed for presence of any free fluid in anterior and posterior location, for this one should screen parasternal long-axis (PLAX) and apical region.

EXTENDED FAST

This includes screening of right and left thorax to detect pneumothorax or hemothorax or both (Figs. 11.12A to D).

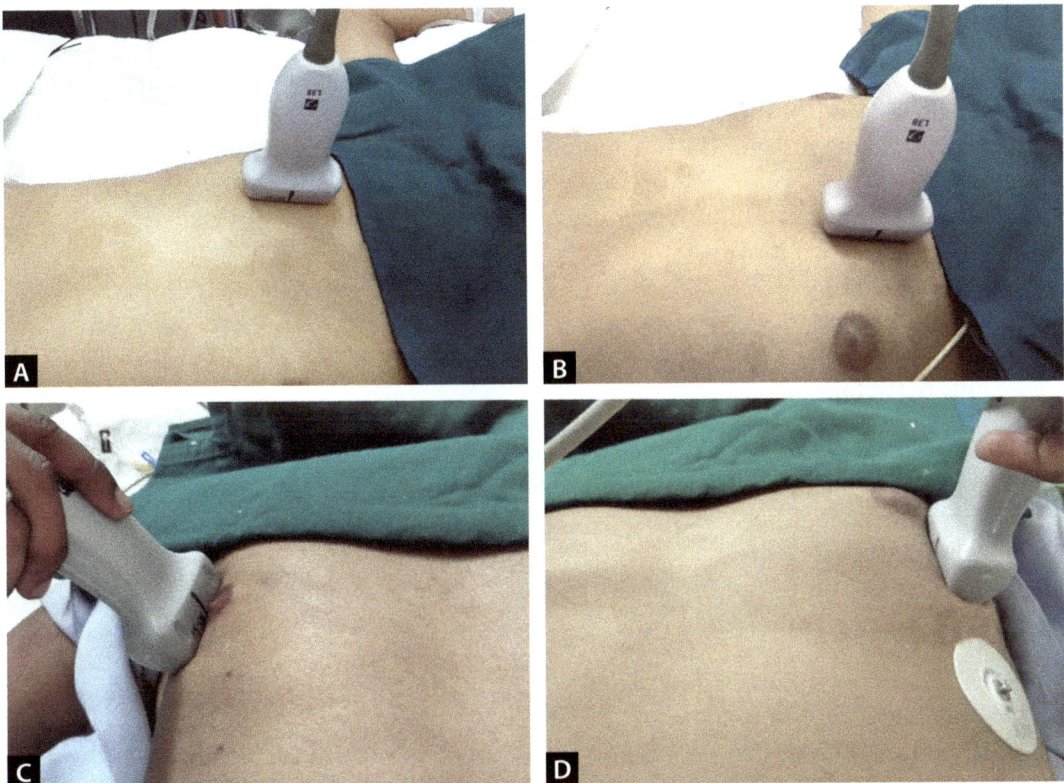

Figs. 11.12A to D: Extended FAST (A) eFAST right parasternal; (B) eFAST left parasternal; (c) eFAST right chest; (d) eFast left chest.

Pneumothorax

Linear probe or curvilinear probe (depth 4 cm).

Probe is placed on anterior chest wall in longitudinal axis with marker dot pointing toward cephalad—just 2–3 cm away from lateral margin of sternum 3rd to 4th intercostal space (both right and left side to be screened).

As collection of air is position dependent other sites should also be screened (details in chapter on lung ultrasound).

Pneumothorax will be seen as absence of lung sliding and bar code in M-mode (details in chapter on lung ultrasound).

Hemothorax

Right Side

In RUQ view, slide the probe cephalad to obtain view of diaphragm. Blood or fluid appears as jet black triangle just superior to diaphragm.

Left Side

In LUQ view, rotate the probe clockwise so that the marker dot points toward posterior axilla, diaphragm is seen just superior to spleen. Pleural collection will appear as jet black stripe or just superior to diaphragm. USG in trauma can also give significant information in following injuries:

Ultrasonography in trauma can also give us information about:
- Musculoskeletal injuries
- Fractures
- Foreign body
- Neurotrauma
- Optic nerve injury.

Musculoskeletal injuries: With advent of high resolution ultrasound imaging musculoskeletal imaging can be obtained at par with magnetic resonance imaging (MRI), which was the main modality earlier.
- Technical considerations
- High frequency linear probe is preferred to image musculotendinous structures
- Water bath or standoff pad is used.

Normal look of musculoskeletal structures:
- *Skin*: Thin hyperechoic at the top.
- *Subcutaneous layer:* Reticular appearance due to fat which varies in thickness according to body mass index.
- *Muscle*:
    - *Longitudinal view:* Hypoechoic appearance with hyperechoic striations.
    - *Transverse view:* Speckled appearance.
- *Fascial layers*: Thin and intensely hyperechoic following muscle.
- *Tendons*: Longitudinal view—hyperechoic and linear.
- *Transverse view:* Moderate echogenicity with hyperechoic bundles.
- Anisotropy.
- *Bone* has intensely hyperechoic rim with posterior shadows.

Neurovascular bundle: Artery and vein appears as an as anechoic structures and nerve as hyperechoic with grapelike structures.

The entire muscle at the site of impact should be studied, paying particular attention to surrounding structures to rule out compression and vascular damage.
- Injuries may be seen *as hypoechoic* focal lesion in mild injury to fraying of muscle fibers in moderate injury to hematoma along with above findings in severe injury.
- Hematoma is seen as inhomogeneous mass which may be intramuscular, extramuscular localized or extending along the fascia or spreading to subcutaneous tissue or down to bone.
- Appearance also vary on time elapsed. Within first 24 hours may appear both hypoechoic and hyperechoic and later hypoechoic to anechoic.

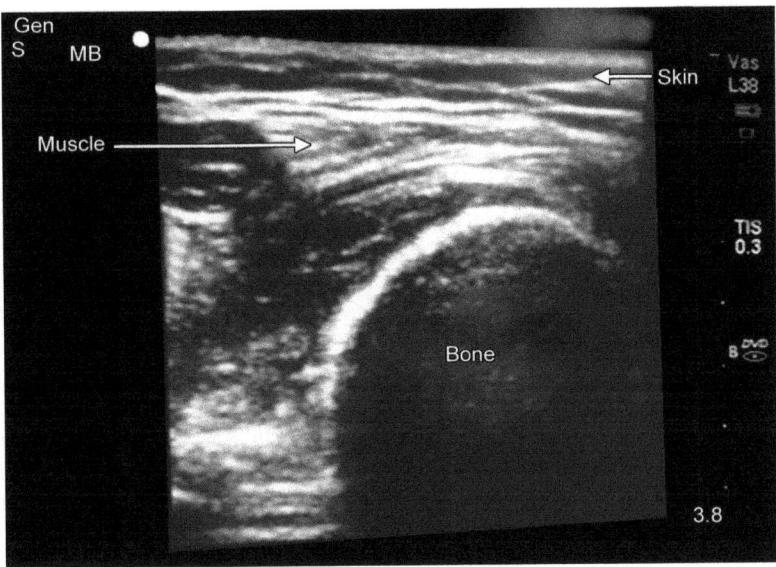

Fig. 11.13: USG showing appearance of bony structures.

- Thus, US examination aids in:
  - Correct assessment of severity of injuries
  - Location of extension of the lesion
  - To assess possible compression of surrounding structures.

Fracture: The interface of relatively hypoechoic soft tissue to hyperechoic cortex of bone makes an ideal condition for detection of fractures by ultrasound (Fig. 11.13).

Probe: Linear array transducer with generous amount of gel.

Technique: Examination is started by placing probe on point of maximum tenderness.

It may be painful so patient should be counseled and care should be taken while applying pressure at fracture site.

Ribs: The bone image appears as a hyperechoic semicircle and just deep to ribs pleural line can be seen with comets or B, lines. Once disruptions is seen, rib should be imaged in longitudinal plane, the angulation of rib should be kept in mind and probe position should be adjusted accordingly.

Rib fracture appears as discontinuation in anterior cortex of bone and a small hematoma may be seen surrounding fracture site, once rib fracture is seen one should rule out pneumothorax (Fig. 11.14).

Nasal fracture: Linear probe is placed on lateral pyramids (both sides) and paramedially and medially to evaluate the bone fully.

As nasal bones are superficial, depth should be adjusted accordingly.

Fracture area will be hypoechoic and may be surrounded by hematoma.

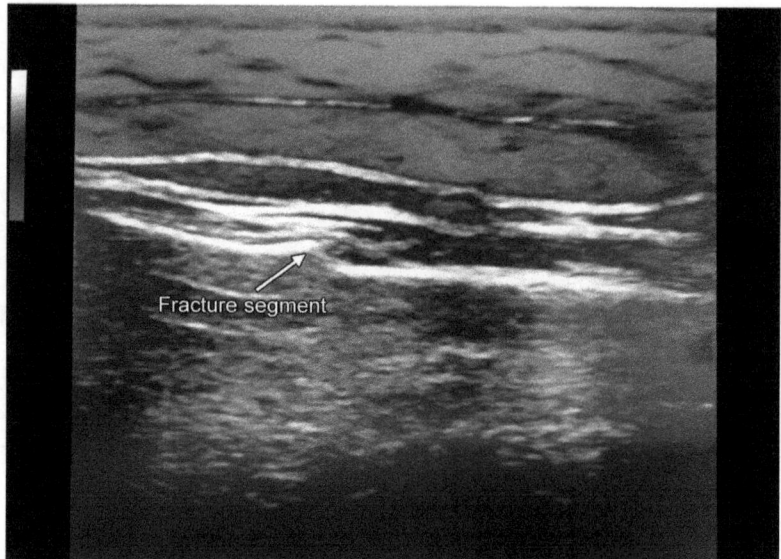

Fig. 11.14: RIB fractures, note breach in cortex.

Long bone fractures: They are seen as disruption in cortical surface with surrounding hematoma.

Hyoid bone: Fracture of hyoid bone will be seen as disruption of hyperechoic cortex with a step off like pattern.

Foreign body: Foreign body (FB) are quite often missed on routine examination and may face medicolegal litigation.
- Ultrasound has now become modality of choice for detecting location and removal of foreign body.
- Provider should have proper knowledge of anatomy and neurovascular structures nearby FB.
- *Appearance:* They have variety in appearances and images produced.
- Wood appears as hyperechoic small posterior shadow in transverse view and this shadow may not be seen in longitudinal view.
- Metal will be seen as hyperechoic with reverberation.
- Most of them will have surrounding hypoechoic area that is due to edema or cellulitis and or hematoma
- Once located, US helps in removal of FB.

Neurotrauma: It is used mainly to assess midline shift.
- Mainly as an adjunct to CT scan and follow-up
- *Transcranial Doppler:* It measures systolic diastolic and mean arterial pressures and gives us idea about cerebral blood flow.

Note: Most important is to document all findings so that we can compare.

SUGGESTED READING

1. Bowra J, McLaughlin RE. FAST and EFAST. Emergency Ultrasound Made Easy, Second edition; 2011.
2. ED Course manual 2 EFAST by Dr Justin Bowra The San Emergency Ultrasound Manual.
3. GS Rozycki. Surgical clinics of North America. Abdominal ultrasonography in trauma 1995. Elsevier volume 75 issue 2 april 1995; pp. 175 – 91.
4. Haung M, et al. Ultrasonography for evaluation of hemoperitoneal during resuscitation: a simple scoring system trauma. 1994;36:173-7.
5. Mckenney, et al. Sonography as a primary screening technique for blunt abdominal trauma. AJR Am J Ronentgenol. 1998;170:979-85.
6. Rippey JCR, Royse AG. Ultrasound in trauma. Best Pract Res Clin Anaesthesiol 2009; 23: 343–62.
7. Robert Reardon. Sonoguide [Ultrasound guide for Emergency Physicians: Ultrasound in trauma-fast examination AIUM [American Institute of Ultrasound in Medicine] 2014 : Focused examination with Sonography [FAST] Examination, parameter developed in collaboration with the American College of Emergency Physicians. Journal of Ultrasound 2013; 16(4);209 – 14.
8. SIRLIN Claude B, et al. Quantification of fluid on screening ultrasonography for blunt abdominal trauma: a simple scoring system to predict severity of injury ultrasound medicine 2001;20:359–64.

CHAPTER 12

Ultrasound-guided Vascular Access

Sachin Jagdale

INTRODUCTION

Vascular access is an integral part of patient care. Access may be needed for diagnostic or therapeutic procedures. Vascular access may be challenging and technically difficult by conventional method for various reasons like abnormal anatomy, coagulopathy, obesity, thrombosed veins, etc.

Ultrasound (US)-guided procedures in such cases enable accurate location of relevant anatomy, increases success rates, are safer and decrease the risk of complications.

Useful when there is difficulty in obtaining peripheral intravascular (IV) access by traditional means due to edema, dark skin, etc.

ADVANTAGES

Decreases the risk associated with conventional (landmark) technique.

Trials and observation studies have found that US-guided cannulation decreases time to cannulation and risks of complications.
- Faster access
- Fewer attempts
- High success rates
- Lower complication rates
- Can confirm position of guidewire in target vessel.

EQUIPMENT

1. *Transducer used*: Linear transducer with higher frequency (7–12 MHz) and higher resolution for superficial structures (Fig. 12.1).
2. Sterility must be maintained during procedure. Sterile probe covers/sterile gloves (Fig. 12.2).
3. Sterile gels/antiseptic solution can be used as scanning medium (Fig. 12.3).

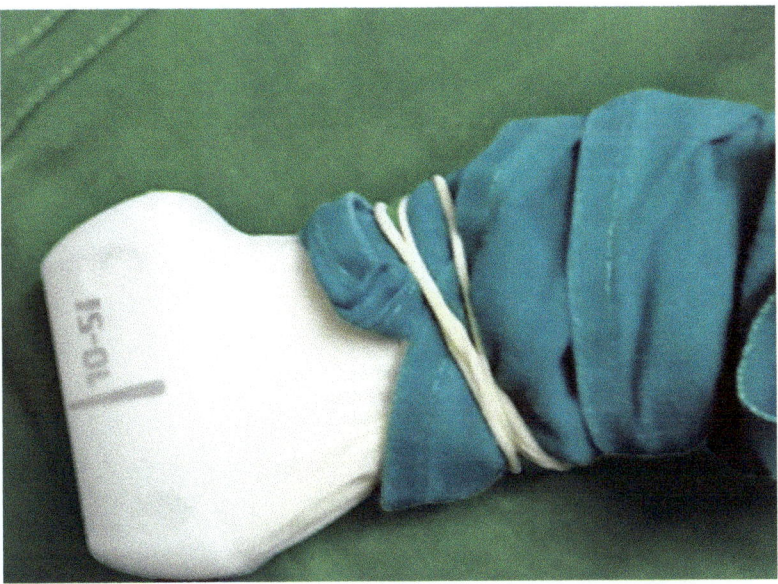

Fig. 12.1: Linear transducer.

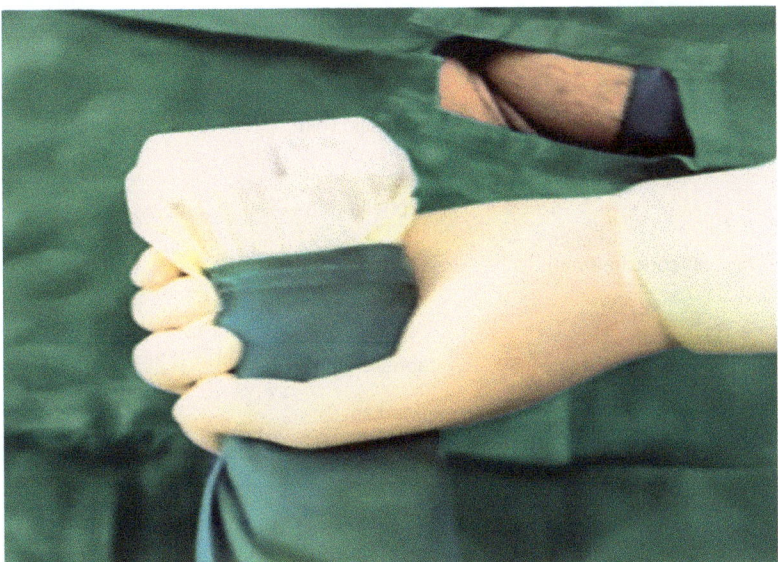

Fig. 12.2: Linear transducer covered with sterile glove and sterile dressing.

ANATOMY OF COMMONLY ACCESSED VESSELS

1. *Dorsal venous arch*:
   - Network of veins on dorsum of hand which receives tributaries from fingers and palms
   - It drains into cephalic and basilic veins (Fig. 12.4).

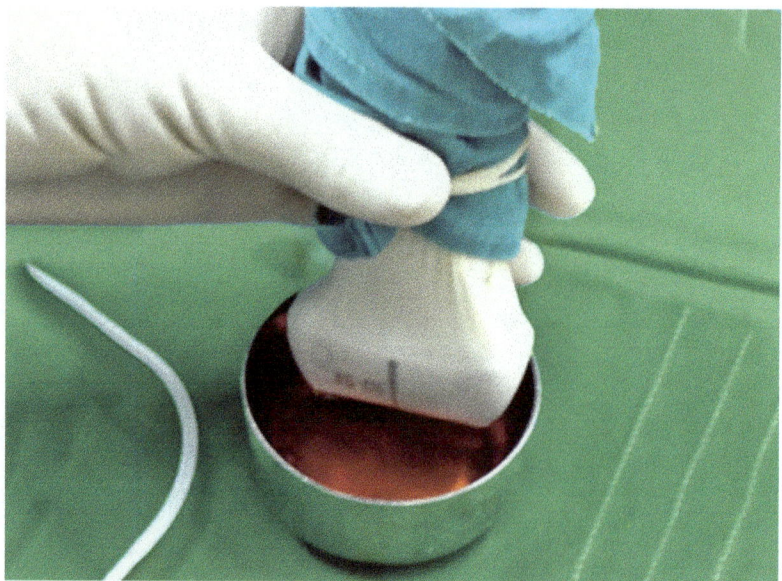

Fig. 12.3: Solution used as scanning medium.

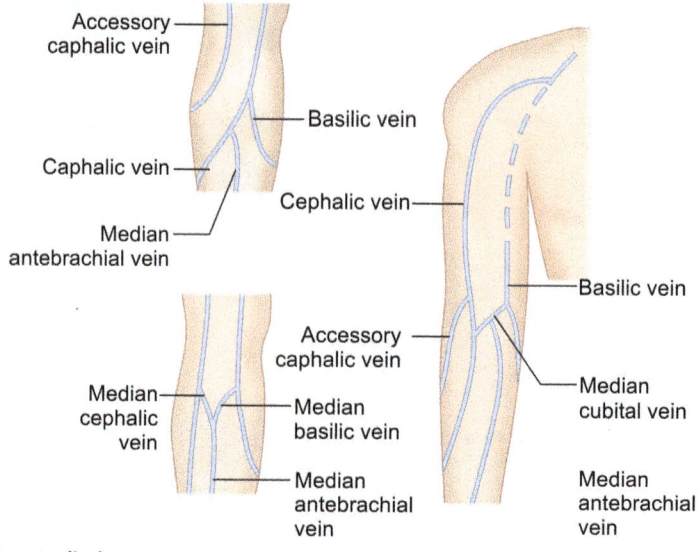

Fig. 12.4: Veins of upper limb.

2. *Cephalic vein*:
   - Begins at lateral border of venous arch
   - It ascends on radial border of forearm and continues upward in front of elbow and upward in arm around lateral border of biceps (Fig. 12.4)
   - And further upward where it drains in axillary vein.

3. *Basilic vein*:
   - Continuation of medial border of venous arch
   - Runs upward along medial border of forearm, continues upward in front of elbow along medial side of biceps
   - Unites further with brachial vein to form axillary vein which continues as axillary vein and then subclavian vein.
4. *Subclavian vein*:
   - It is continuation of axillary vein and runs from outer border of first rib to medial border of anterior scalene muscle where it joins internal jugular vein (IJV) to form brachiocephalic vein (innominate vein) (Fig. 12.5)
   - Subclavian vein lies anterior to anterior scalene muscle while subclavian artery lies posterior to anterior scalene muscle.
5. *Internal jugular vein*:
   - Internal jugular vein runs in carotid sheath usually lateral to common carotid artery (CCA) and deep to sternocleidomastoid muscle from base of skull anteriorly toward sternum.
6. *External jugular vein*:
   - Formed by union of retromandibular vein and posterior auricular vein and runs down perpendicularly from angle of mandible toward mid-clavicle where it pierces deep fascia and joins subclavian vein.
7. *Femoral vein and artery*:
   - Femoral vein accompanies femoral artery in femoral sheath. It begins at adductor canal (Hunter's canal) and ends at inferior margin of inguinal ligament (Fig. 12.6)

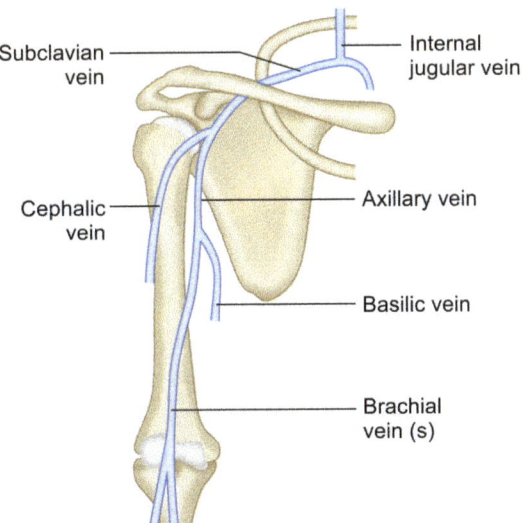

Fig. 12.5: Major veins of neck and upper limb.

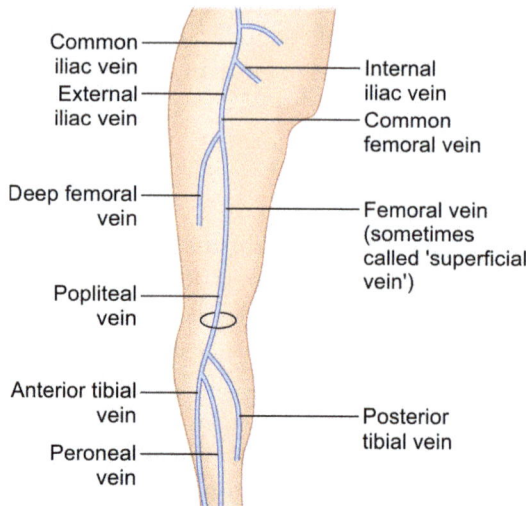

Fig. 12.6: Deep veins of lower limb.

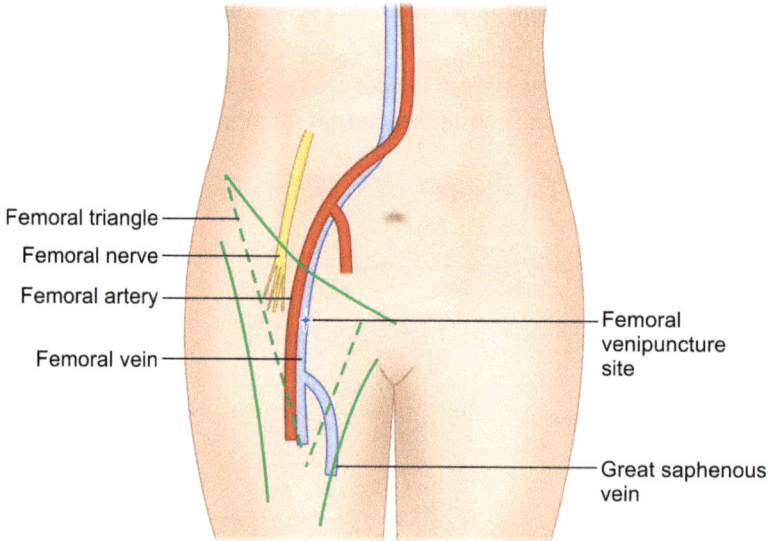

Fig. 12.7: "Femoral triangle"—femoral artery, vein and nerve.

- In femoral triangle, vein is medial to femoral artery (Fig. 12.7)
- Vein → Artery → Nerve (medial to lateral)
- In short axis (SAX) view, common femoral artery (CFA), femoral vein and great saphenous vein (GSV) appear like famous cartoon character "Mickey Mouse" (Fig. 12.8).

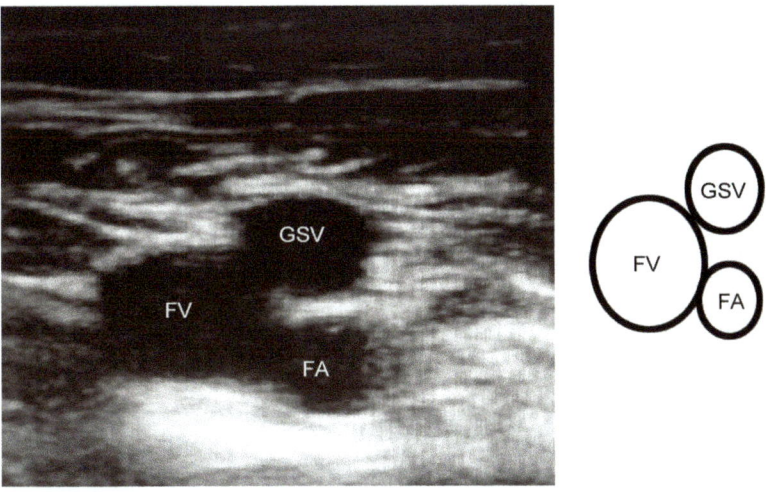

Fig. 12.8: "Mickey Mouse sign"—short axis view showing Mickey Mouse-shaped image formed by femoral artery (FA), femoral vein (FV), great saphenous vein (GSV).

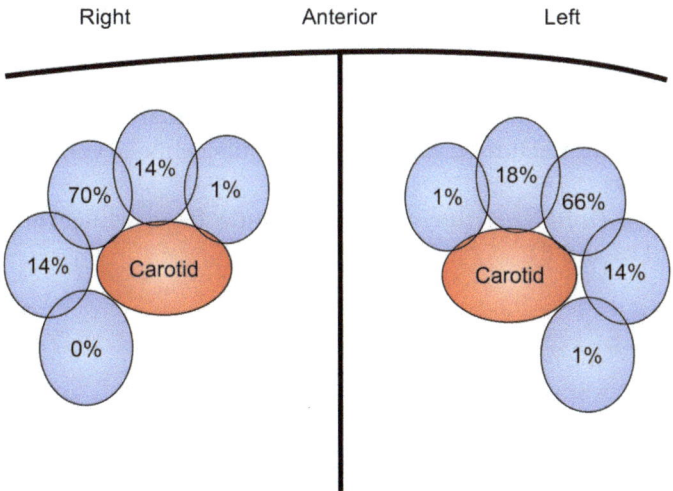

Fig. 12.9: Anatomic variations of internal jugular vein (IJV) to carotid artery (CA).

- Anatomic variation of IJV relative to carotid artery (Fig. 12.9)
- Similarly anatomic variations can be seen in other blood vessels.
8. *Commonly accessed arteries*:
    - Radial artery, ulnar artery, brachial artery, axillary artery, femoral artery and dorsalis pedis artery.

The technique of US-guided cannulation remains unchanged.

Before proceeding with radial artery cannulation, modified Allen test is performed to confirm collateral supply of blood.

Modified Allen test:
- Hand is elevated and patient is asked to clench fist for 30 seconds
- Pressure is applied over both, radial and ulnar arteries to occlude them
- The hand is then opened and appears blanched or pale.
- Ulnar pressure is released and color change should occur in 5–15 seconds
- Means Allen test is negative (normal).

DIFFERENTIATING ARTERY FROM VEIN

- Arteries and veins appear anechoic (black)
- Arterial margins are brighter with thicker wall, are round, pulsatile, and less compressible.
- Veins have thin walls, are oval in shape, easily compressible and nonpulsatile (Figs. 12.10A and B).
- Veins are usually larger in diameter than artery.
- Vein diameter changes with Valsalva maneuver and with respiration.
- Doppler helps in differentiating in difficult cases:
  - *Color Doppler*: Arteries appear red and veins appear blue
  - Mnemonic B-A-R-T (Blue Away, Red Toward) helps to differentiate artery versus vein
  - Assignment of color frequency shifts is usually based on directions (e.g. red for Doppler shifts toward US probe and blue for shifts away from it)
  - Flow within arterial lumen will appear pulsatile; while in vein will be constant rumble of color flow
  - *Pulse wave Doppler*: Arteries have pulsatile flow, while veins have phasic flow (Figs. 12.11A and B).

PROCEDURE/TECHNIQUE OF ULTRASOUND-GUIDED CANNULATION

- Prescan—the area and vessel of interest
- Prepare—for the procedure
- Procedure

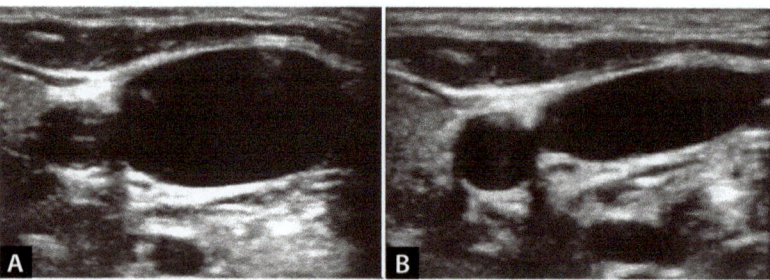

Figs. 12.10A and B: Veins have thin walls, larger and oval in shape and easily compressible.

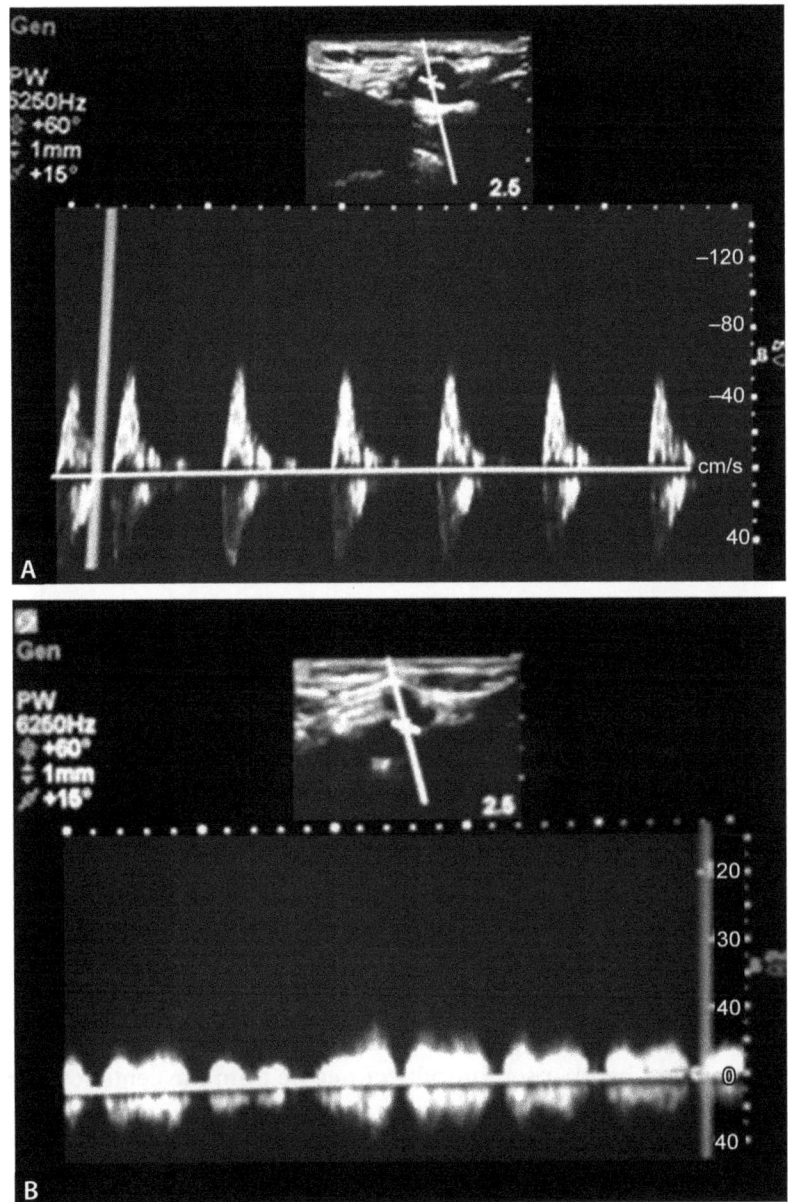

Figs. 12.11A and B: (A) Artery—pulsatile flow; (B) Veins—phasic flow.

- Postscan—confirm guidewire in vessel lumen and screening for complications like hematoma, pneumothorax/hemothorax, etc.

Injection of agitated saline can also be used to produce hyperechoic contrast within lumen of vessel.

Static Technique

- Prescan and identify the target vessel, confirm depth, patency and course of the vessel.
- Mark the site of needle entry and course of vessel.
- Make sure patient does not move or change the position.
- Universal sterile precautions and proceed as in conventional technique.

Advantages

- Technically less demanding and sterilization of probe is not required.

Disadvantage

- Not as safe as real-time US-guided technique.

Dynamic or Real-Time Technique

Out of Plane/Short Axis/Transverse Technique

- *Prescan*:
  - Prescan the area and the vessel of interest
  - Apt patient position, e.g. Trendelenburg position for IJV with neck rotated to contralateral side, leg abduction for femoral cannulation and hand abduction with tourniquet application for peripheral vascular applications.
- *Prepare*:
  - Universal sterile precautions to be taken
  - Ultrasound monitor in your line of sight (Fig. 12.12)
  - Confirm probe marker and marker on monitor to be on same side.
- *Procedure*:
  - Place the probe (US beam) perpendicular to target vessel with nondominant hand
  - Identify the structures and confirm the vessel
  - Move the probe to bring target vessel in center of screen
  - With dominant hand, insert introducer needle from the center of probe at a steeper angle under real-time visualization
  - The image of needle is not seen but a "ring down" artifact is seen where US plane intersects needle
  - Advance the needle slowly, watch for "tenting" of vein wall inward as needle approaches the vessel (Fig. 12.13)
  - The wall bounces back as the vessel is entered
  - The needle tip in the vessel gives an appearance like "bulls eye" or "target sign" (hyperechoic needle in center of anechoic vessel) (Figs. 12.14 and 12.15)
  - Confirm by aspirating blood and introduce guidewire.

Ultrasound-guided Vascular Access

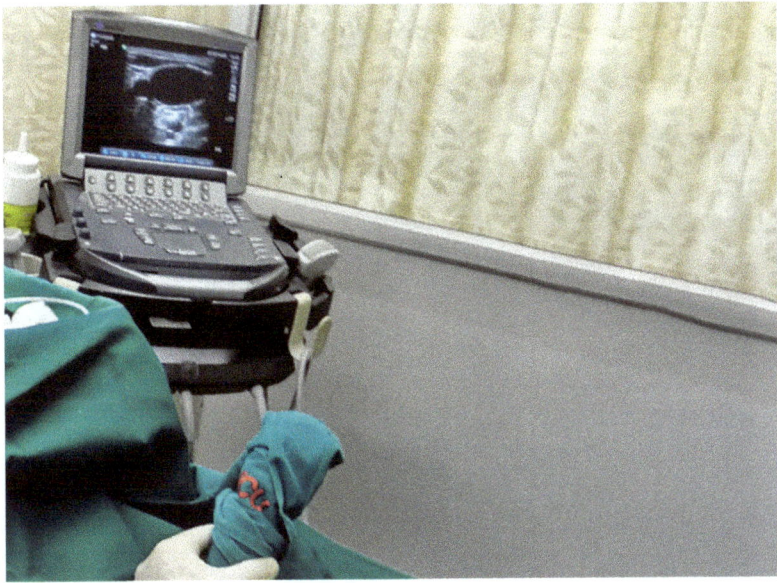

Fig. 12.12: Ultrasound monitor in line of sight, confirm marker on probe and monitor beyond same side.

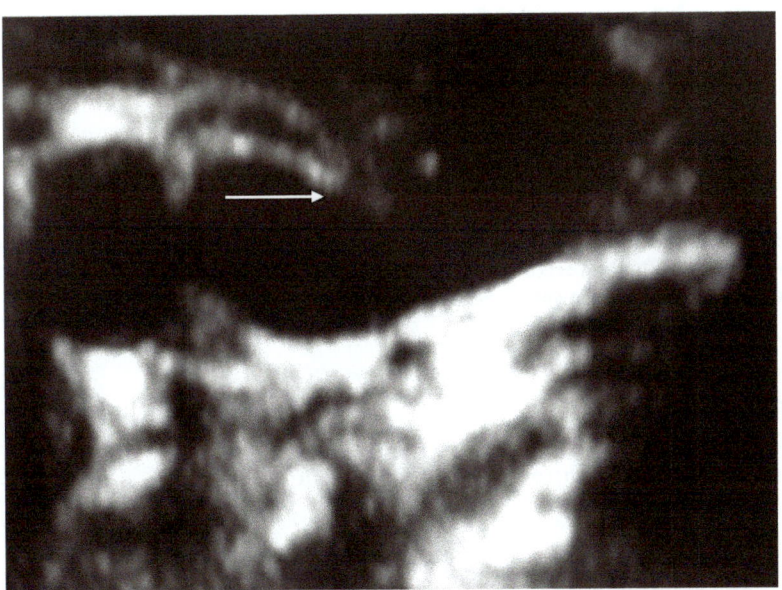

Fig. 12.13: "Tenting" of vein wall.

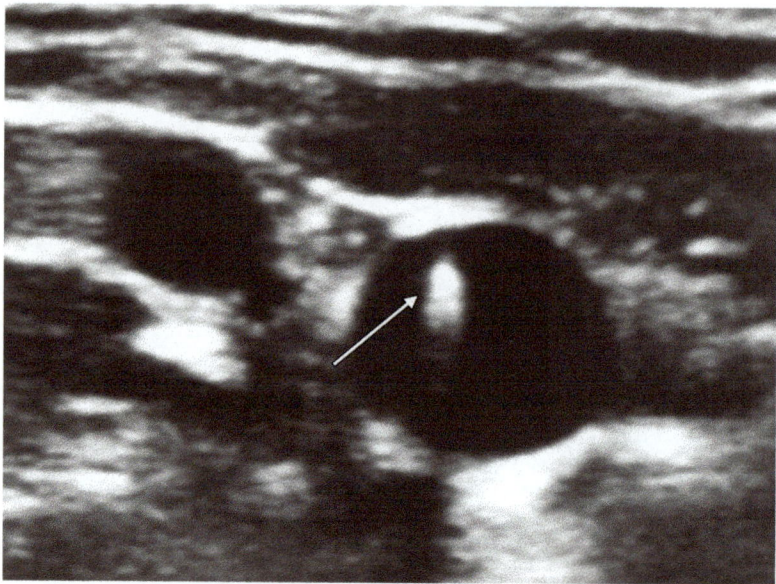

Fig. 12.14: "Bulls eye" or "target sign".

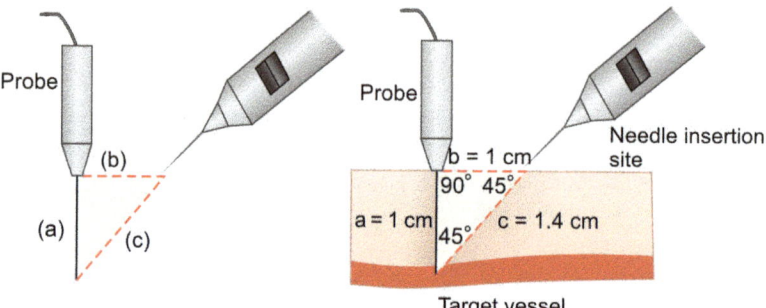

Fig. 12.15: Short axis technique. Measure depth of vessel from center of probe and if needle entry site from probe is same as the depth, then according to Pythagoras theorem the distance traveled by needle will be 1.4 times the depth, provided needle entry angle is 45°.

- *Postscan*:
  – Guidewire should be visible in vessel lumen
  – Complete the procedure by Seldinger technique.

Advantages

- Better lateral resolution and easier to learn.

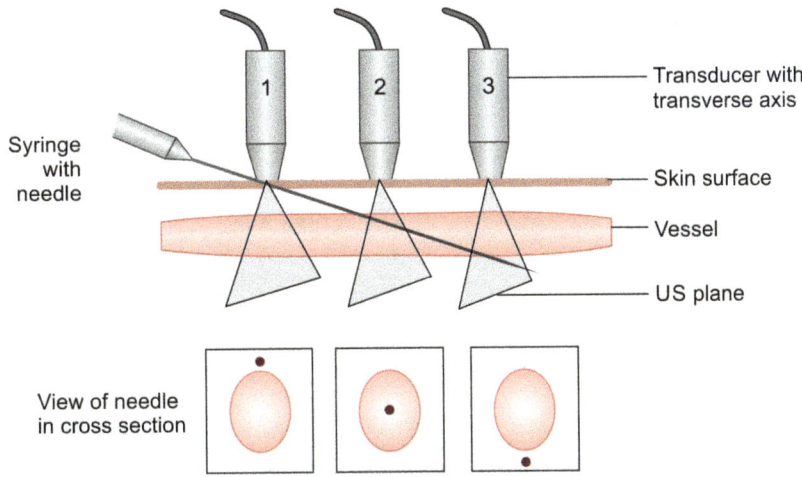

Fig. 12.16: Short axis view. Even though the needle has gone entirely through the vessel, depending on the probe position, it will appear to be proximal in position 1, within the vessel lumen in position 2, and beyond the vessel in position 3.

Disadvantages

- Entire needle cannot be seen and only "ring down" artifact is seen, hence the risk of overshoot or "through-and-through" puncture (Fig. 12.16).

In-Plane/Long Axis/Longitudinal Technique

- Prescan and preparation is same as for out of plane technique.
- *Procedure*:
  - Identify the target vessel in transverse scan
  - Turn US probe parallel to target vessel (longitudinal plane)
  - Hold the probe with nondominant hand in longitudinal plane
  - Ensure probe pointer is toward piercing end
  - Insert the introducer needle at a shallow angle (30°) from center of probe in longitudinal plane
  - Needle will be seen entering from left on the screen
  - Aspirate and advance the needle till needle is seen entering the vessel
  - Entire needle can be seen on screen if US beam and needle are in same plane
  - Confirm by aspirating blood and introduce guidewire.
- *Postscan*:
  - Confirm guidewire position in the vessel and complete the procedure using Seldinger technique.

Advantages:
- Entire needle path, entry into the vein and passage of guidewire can be seen and confirmed, hence less risk of overshoot (Figs. 12.17 and 12.18).

Disadvantages:
- Poor lateral resolution and technically more challenging.

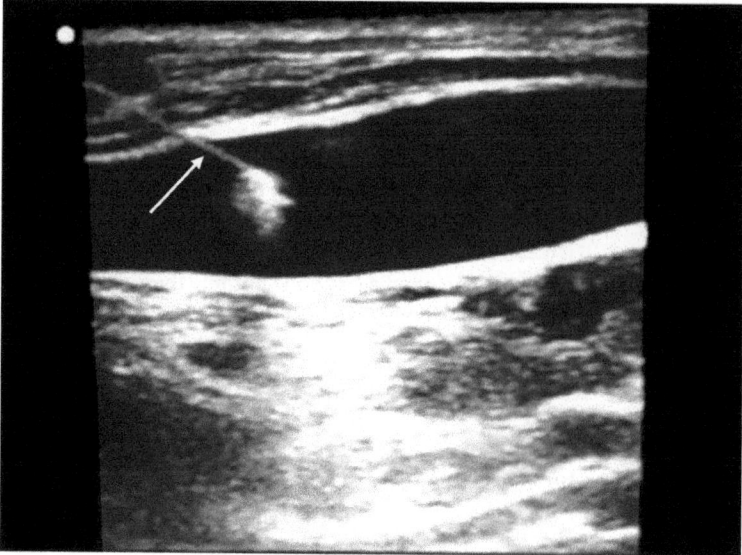

Fig. 12.17: Long axis view. Entire needle path seen with tip in vessel lumen.

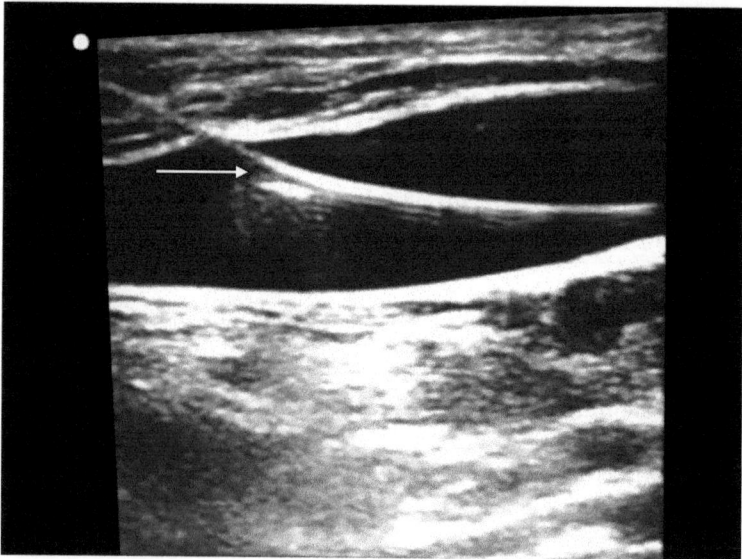

Fig. 12.18: Long axis view. Entire needle seen with guidewire in vessel lumen.

NEWER TECHNIQUES

1. *Wire-in-needle (WIN) technique*:
   - A new US-guided vascular access technique where the needle preloaded with guidewire is used (without the use of syringe)
   - Insertion of needle preloaded with guidewire is performed using long axis (LAX) technique under dynamic US guidance.
2. *Lateral in-plane technique*:
   - Vessel is visualized in SAX and needle is introduced in plane from lateral side of transducer.

COMPARISON BETWEEN LANDMARK TECHNIQUE AND ULTRASOUND-GUIDED TECHNIQUE

Incidence of complications during central venous catheter (CVC) insertion is reported to be 2–15%. Failure rate is approximately 12%.

Various studies have documented that use of real-time US significantly decreases the access time, number of attempts and immediate complications as compared to landmark technique. Even US prescreening and marking to identify the vessel location and patency (static technique) has better results compared to landmark technique.

CONFIRMATION AND DOCUMENTATION

- Confirm guidewire within vessel lumen.
- Injection of agitated saline can also be used to produce hyperechoic contrast.
- Ultrasound can also be used to guide and confirm position of temporary pacing wire.
- Ultrasound image utilized (SAX/LAX), technique used and confirmation of successful cannulation should be documented.

GUIDELINES AND RECOMMENDATIONS

- Suggests two-dimensional (2D) vascular screening prior to cannulation and real-time US needle guidance.
- Can be used for central venous, peripheral venous and arterial cannulation.
- Can be used to check for immediate life-threatening complications after the procedure.
- Standardized training is suggested to improve patient's safety and outcome.
- Catheter placement in:
    - Internal jugular vein: Category A—Level 1
    - Subclavian vein: Category A—Level 3
    - Femoral vein: Category C—Level 2
    - Peripheral venous access: Category B—Level 2
    - Radial artery cannulation: Category A—Level 1.

SUGGESTED READING

1. Bowra J, McLaughlin RE. Emergency Ultrasound Made Easy. Edinburgh: Churchill Livingstone Elsevier; 2011.
2. Lamperti M, Bodenham AR, Pittiruti M, et al. International evidence-based recommendations on ultrasound-guided vascular access. Intensive Care Med. 2012;38(7):1105-17.
3. Miller AH, Roth BA, Mills TJ, et al. Ultrasound guidance versus the landmark technique for the placement of central venous catheters in the emergency department. Acad Emerg Med. 2002;9(8):800-5.
4. Troianos CA, Hartman GS, Glas KE, et al. Guidelines for performing ultrasound guided vascular cannulation: recommendations of the American Society of Echocardiography and the Society of Cardiovascular Anesthesiologists. J Am Soc Echocardiogr. 2011;24(12):1291-318.
5. Wallace BA, Taylor T. (2018). Ultrasound-guided venous access. [online] Available from www.cdemcurriculum.com/ultrasound-guided-venous-access/. [Accessed June, 2018].

14 CHAPTER

Ultrasound-guided Procedures

Kedar Toraskar

INTRODUCTION

Various beside procedures are done on a day-to-day basis in the critical care, emergency departments. Ultrasound is a cost-effective imaging tool to make these procedure safe, successful and effective with fewer complication rates as compared to those without ultrasonography (USG) guidance.

Ultrasonography has been used during the last 50 years to aid in diagnosis and guide procedures.[1]

Most of the procedural guidelines are moving towards adopting USG guidance as an integral part of these procedures which will be the norm of the future. In this review we will be reviewing a few procedures commonly done in the critical care and emergency departments along with general principles guiding them. The salient points of the following USG guided procedures will be discussed.

ASPIRATION

- Thoracocentesis/pericardiocentesis/paracentesis
- Transvenous and transcutaneous pacing
- Percutaneous tracheostomy and cricothyrotomy
- Lumbar puncture.

WHY USG FOR PROCEDURES?

It allows visualization of anatomy prior to an invasive procedure and thereby detects abnormal anatomy, identifies interposed structures and gives a better localizing of the target. More importantly it can prevent an invasive procedure being attempted when not indicated.

Point-of-care ultrasound is especially important during deep-needle procedures such as central line insertion because the provider can visualize the needle in a dynamic, real-time fashion. Such technology has enabled health care providers to achieve a high degree of first-pass success and has decreased complications when compared with traditional, landmark-based approaches.[2]

CHOICE OF PROBE

The linear or high frequency probe 5–13 MHz for superficial targets and the curvilinear or low frequency probe 2–5 MHz for deeper targets. The phased array or cardiac probe can be used for cardiac interventional procedures like pacing and pericardiocentesis.

ULTRASOUND IMAGE

Fluid is black, soft tissues are gray, air and metal are hyperechoic and cause reverberation while bone and stones cause shadowing.

In transverse plane, the needle casts a comet tail and beam width artefact while a reverberation (ring down) artefact is seen in the longitudinal plane. Size and depth measurement along with the angle of needle entry on the USG image is very important for any successful procedure. Two methods namely indirect or static method and direct or real time methods are used for performing any USG guided procedures.

Indirect or Static Method

This method is best suited for large static targets, e.g. ascites, pleural effusion which are not too far away from the skin or small superficial targets.

Steps Involved

First locate target with ultrasound (US) and identify best site for skin entry. Then measure size, depth and observe for changes with respiration. Then note midpoint in the axial direction of transducer followed by removal of the transducer marking the skin and performing the procedure.

Advantages
It is easy with less coordination and less experience required with no requirement for sterile transducer cover.

Direct Method

Needle is advanced under direct ultrasound vision. This method has a transverse (out of plane) and longitudinal (in plane) approach.

Transverse Approach

In this approach the target is in center of image and the needle approach is perpendicular to the scan plane.

Advantages: It requires less space at the anatomical site and one can avoid structures on either side of the target using a steeper angle of approach.

Disadvantages: The needle is harder to see in cross section and the depth of the needle is difficult to assess so one has to rely on just the tissue movement. Also a sterile transducer cover is required.

Longitudinal Approach

The target is in the longitudinal section across image and needle approach is along the scan plane.

Advantages: Better localization of needle which is visually striking and the needle can be seen all the way to the target. Also the structures deep and superficial to the target can be clearly seen.

Disadvantages: It is difficult to line up three objects, i.e. the ultrasound beam, needle and the target. It requires more coordination and practice. One cannot see structures either side of target and two adjacent parallel structures can look similar so it is easy to slip from one to the other. Also more space is required at anatomical site.

General principles for USG procedures:
- Ensure patient and operator comfort
- Line up the patient, target and transducer, and screen
- Watch the screen not your hands
- Use the transducer to find the needle
- Make sure local anesthetic is free of air
- Do not compromise on aseptic precautions and probe sterility (Fig. 14.1)
- Do not undermine the landmarks but respect them.

ULTRASOUND-GUIDED PARACENTESIS

Paracentesis is a deep needle procedure that has both diagnostic and therapeutic indications. The procedure can help identify the presence of infection or the cause of new-onset ascites.

The mechanical complications of a paracentesis are relatively rare, but when they occur, they can have significant morbidity and mortality. Intraperitoneal hemorrhage, abdominal wall hematomas, bowel perforation, and bladder perforation have been reported with the traditional procedure.

Fortunately, point-of-care ultrasound is a very sensitive tool for identification of fluid within the peritoneal cavity and can also distinguish structural impediments to the safe introduction of a paracentesis needle, such as the bladder, bowel, solid organs, and pregnant uterus (Fig. 14.2).[3]

Ultrasound assistance displays the largest pocket of readily accessible fluid and will identify the presence of fluid mimics, such as a cystic mass or ventral hernia. Furthermore, in a prospective, randomized study comparing point-of-care ultrasound guidance with the traditional technique, operators increased their success rate from 65% to 95% when using ultrasound assistance.[4]

Ultrasound-guided Procedures

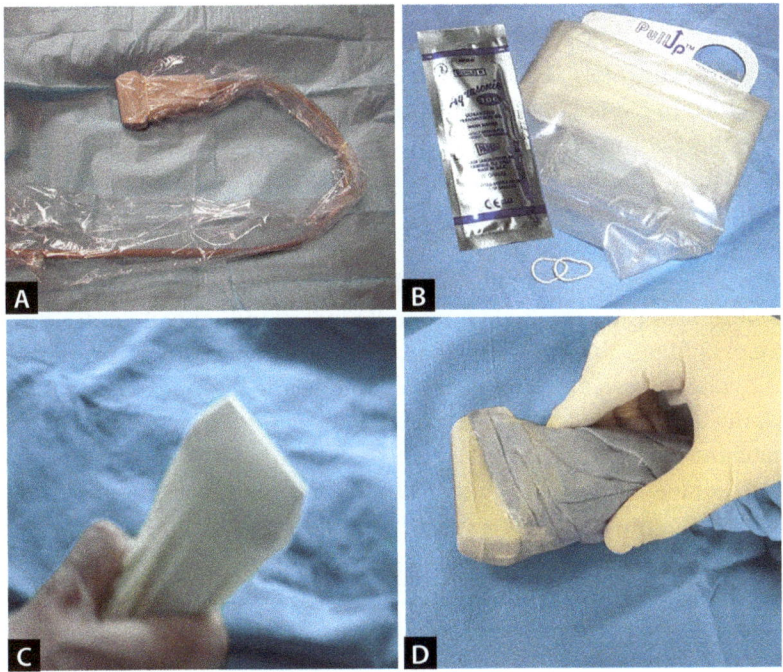

Fig. 14.1: Different methods of probe sterilization.

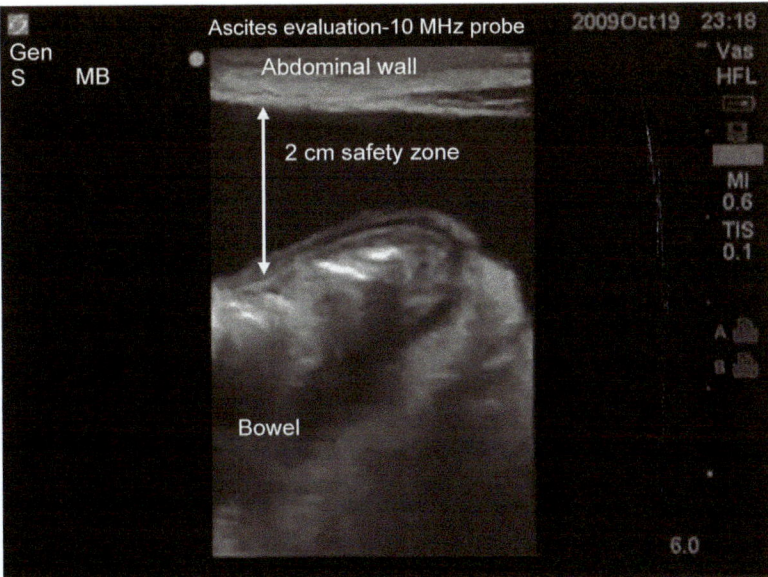

Fig. 14.2: Ultrasound-guided paracentesis (safety zone).

ULTRASOUND-GUIDED THORACENTESIS

Ultrasonography improves the accuracy of site selection for needle insertion, thereby improving safety and increasing the likelihood of a successful procedure.[5] Ultrasound should guide the selection of the puncture site by identifying an intercostal space with underlying pleural fluid that is of sufficient depth that the lung will not be pierced by the needle during aspiration (typically >10 mm) (Fig. 14.3).

Once the intercostal space is chosen, the needle insertion site is marked using firm indentation with a needle cap. Following the identification of the needle insertion site, the examiner determines the best angle for needle insertion that will access the fluid and avoid adjacent organs. Ideally, this is achieved by selecting an angle that is perpendicular to the skin surface, which is easier to duplicate with the needle/syringe assembly. Once the angle is determined, the depth for needle penetration is measured from a frozen image on the screen using the machine caliper function.

Following thoracentesis, the ipsilateral chest is examined for pneumothorax by ultrasound and findings documented. The presence of lung sliding at multiple interspaces is a sensitive finding that rules out a procedure-related pneumothorax. Several nonrandomized studies demonstrate that use of ultrasound guidance in non-ventilated patients reduce the rate of pneumothorax following thoracentesis to less than 3% when performed by adequately trained operators.[6]

In a prospective study, ultrasound guidance increased the rate of accurate puncture sites by 26% and prevented possible accidental organ puncture in 10% of all cases within the study. The rates of dry punctures and number of attempts were also shown to decrease, which may decrease patient discomfort.

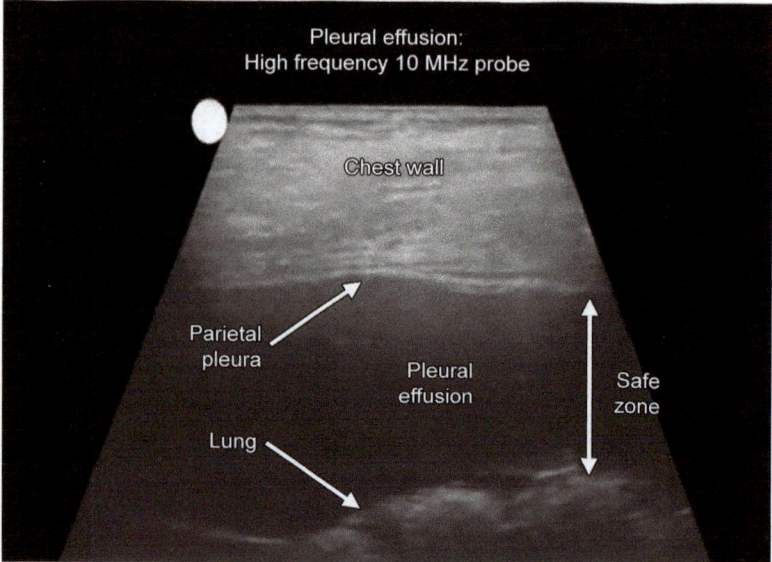

Fig. 14.3: Safe zone for thoracentesis with USG guidance.

ULTRASOUND-GUIDED PERICARDIOCENTESIS

Ultrasound remains the principal diagnostic test to confirm critical pericardial effusion and should always be used to guide aspiration when available. In contrast to the high rates of procedure-related complications associated with blind aspiration,[7] multiple observational studies of ultrasound-guided pericardiocentesis report improved safety, clinician satisfaction and success (greater than 97%)

One of three techniques may be employed for ultrasound-guided pericardiocentesis:
1. Static imaging uses ultrasound guidance for procedure planning, but does not provide real-time ultrasound imaging during the procedure.
2. Remote guidance uses ultrasound to view the heart and effusion during the procedure but rarely provides direct observation of needle penetration.
3. Dynamic guidance uses real time ultrasound imagery to view and guide the needle during the approach and pericardial puncture.

Using ultrasound, determine the presence and distribution of pericardial fluid. Systematically examine the heart and look for effusions at each imaging window (subcostal, parasternal, apical, and any additional views) (Fig. 14.4). Select the best entry site. This site contains the largest pericardial fluid accumulation that is closest to the chest wall and can be entered without puncturing any adjacent vital organs. Relevant vascular structures to avoid, such as the internal mammary arteries, can be located during this evaluation. Select a target fluid layer (distance from pericardium to epicardium) of at least 1 cm to avoid cardiac puncture.

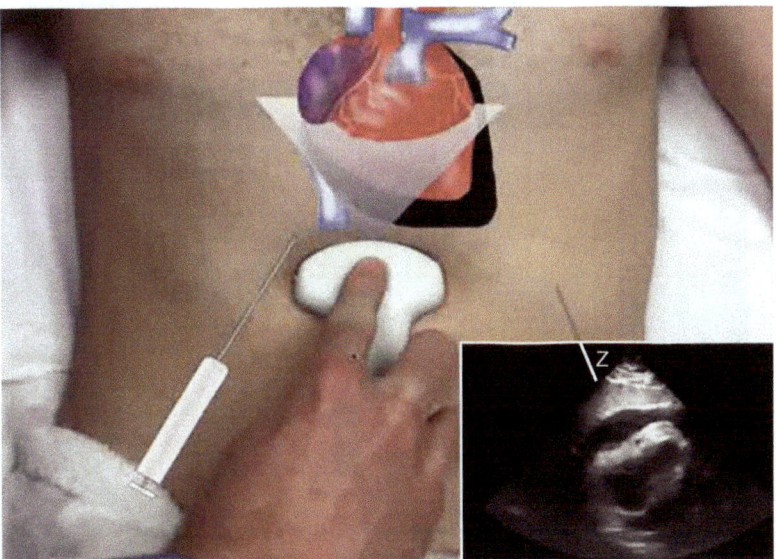

Fig. 14.4: Pericardiocentesis—needle in plane (subcostal approach).

Ultrasound localization of the needle tip may be difficult and bubble contrast injection through the exploring needle is a useful adjunct to confirm needle position. A repeat 2D echo is done after the procedure to quantify the residual fluid and resolution of tamponade.

ULTRASOUND-GUIDED PERCUTANEOUS TRACHEOSTOMY AND CRICOTHYROTOMY

The safety of percutaneous tracheostomy is further increased by using airway USG to delineate the tracheal rings and mark the puncture site between the 2nd and 3rd tracheal rings along with using a bronchoscopic guidance (Fig. 14.5), Airway ultrasound also helps to identify overlying structures like blood vessels and the thyroid isthmus and thereby take pre-emptive measure to avoid them. The same principle holds true for cricothyrotomy. USG helps to accurately identify the trachea in difficult cases where the trachea is not in midline due to pathologies in the neck like goiter and other tumors.

ULTRASOUND-GUIDED LUMBAR PUNCTURE

This is also suggested for patients who are obese or have difficult anatomy because of prior spine surgery or other reasons (Fig. 14.6). A meta-analysis of 14 randomized trials (1334 patients) that compared lumbar punctures and epidural catheterizations performed with ultrasound to those performed without imaging found that ultrasound guidance reduced the risk of failed and traumatic procedures as well as the number of needle insertions and redirections.[8]

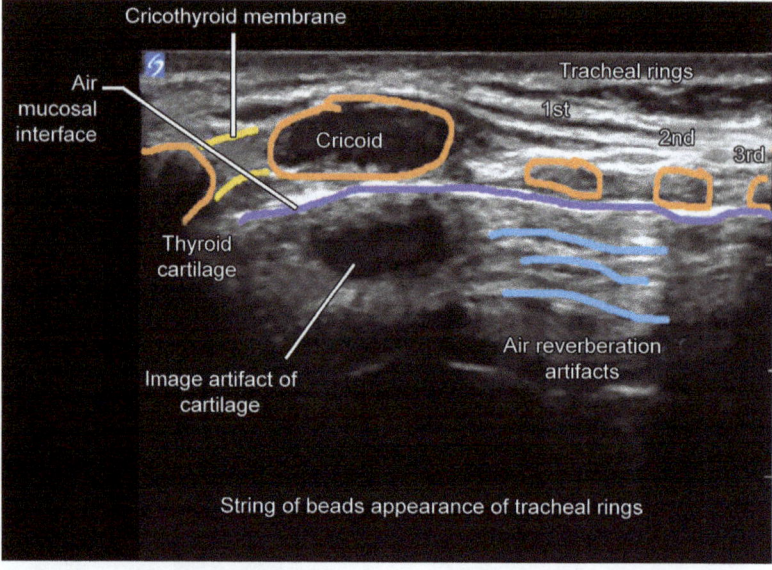

Fig. 14.5: Sagittal plane USG of the airway guided the site of puncture for percutaneous tracheostomy and cricothyrotomy.

ULTRASOUND-GUIDED TRANSVENOUS AND TRANSCUTANEOUS PACING

Ultrasonography is an excellent tool for bedside transvenous pacing along with an electrocardiographic guidance via the bipolar pacing electrode tip which acts as a sensor as well as a pacer. Apart from the operator an additional personnel is required to handle the USG probe to get the 4 chamber subcostal view while guiding the electrode to the right ventricular apex (Fig. 14.7A to C).

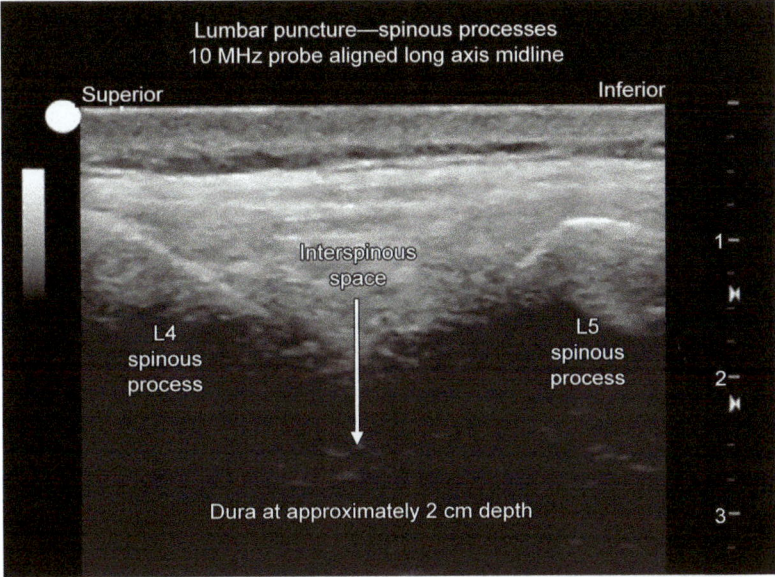

Fig. 14.6: Ultrasound-guided lumbar puncture.

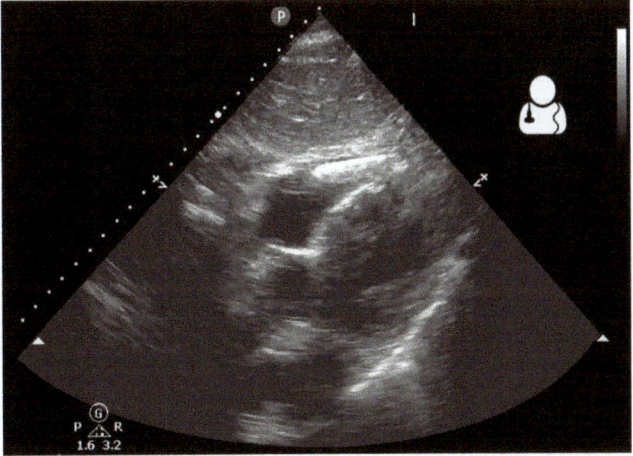

Fig. 14.7A:

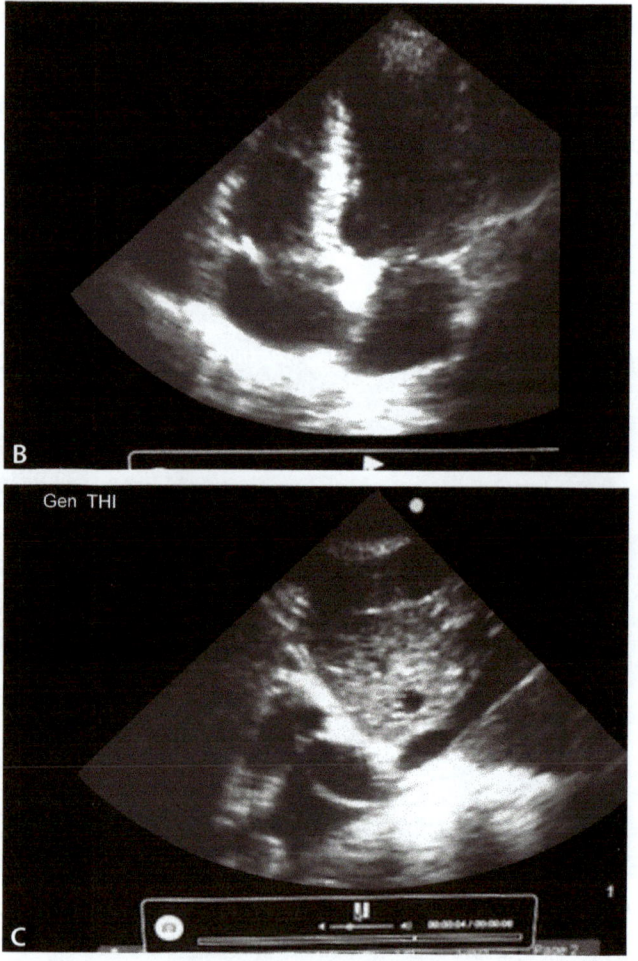

Fig. 14.7B and C:

Fig. 14.7A to C: **(A) Ultrsound- guided transvenous pacing (subcostal 4-chamber view with pacing lead in RV apex); (B) Transvenous pacing wire crossing from RA to RV; (C) Transvenous pacing wire IVC and RA.**

Ultrasonography is also a useful tool to identify true pacing capture during transcutaneous pacing and thereby to optimize the pacing output.

SUMMARY

Ultrasound is useful for many procedures and it improves the safety and success rates of most of the bedside procedures done in the critical care and emergency department. A number of different techniques suit different circumstances hence the basic ultrasound knowledge of the same is required to master the different procedures. Data from survey studies show that there is still a gap between the existing evidence and guidelines and the use of USG in clinical practice. Finally application of the same and practice is required for smooth and successful performance of the above-mentioned procedures.

REFERENCES

1. Nightingale F. Notes on Hospitals; Being Two Papers Read Before the National Association for the Promotion of Social Science, at Liverpool, in October, 1858; With Evidence Given to the Royal Commissioners on the State of the Army in 1857. London, England: Parker; 1859. [Google Scholar]
2. Hind D, Calvert N, McWilliams R, et al. Ultrasonic locating devices for central venous cannulation: meta-analysis. BMJ. 2003;327-61.
3. Butts C. Ultrasound guided procedures. In: Roberts JR, Hedges J (Eds.). Clinical Procedures in Emergency Medicine. 4th edn, Philadelphia, PA: Saunders; 2004: pp.851–6.
4. Mercaldi CJ, Lanes SF. The clinical and economic advantages of ultrasound guidance among patients undergoing paracentesis [abstract]. National Patient Safety Foundation Patient Safety Congress 2011, 2011.
5. Hooper C, Maskell N, BTS audit team, British Thoracic Society national pleural procedures audit 2010, Thorax. 2011;66(7):636-7.
6. Jones PW, Moyers JP, Rogers JT, et al. Ultrasound-guided thoracentesis: is it a safer method? Chest. 2003;123(2):418.
7. Tsang TS, Enriquez-Sarano M, Freeman WK, et al. Consecutive 1127 therapeutic echocardiographically guided pericardiocenteses: clinical profile, practice patterns, and outcomes spanning 21 years. Mayo Clin Proc. 2002;77(5):429.
8. Shaikh F, Brzezinski J, Alexander S, et al. Ultrasound imaging for lumbar punctures and epidural catheterisations: systematic review and meta-analysis. BMJ. 2013;346:f1720. Epub 2013 Mar 26.

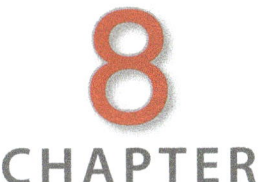

CHAPTER 8

Ultrasound Use in Nephrology, Critical Care Settings and Post-transplant Period

Valentine Lobo, Arindham Kar

INTRODUCTION

A complete abdominal ultrasonography with special reference to the kidneys, ureter and bladder is invaluable as imaging modality while evaluating patients who present as acute kidney injury (AKI). Ultrasonography is noninvasive, and nonnephrotoxic. It can be performed at the bedside unlike a CT scan and provides reasonable diagnostic accuracy in a critically-ill patient. Even in pediatric patients it can be easily performed without the need for sedation unlike CT or MRI. The most important pieces of information obtained from a bedside ultrasonography augmented if necessary by Doppler include (Fig. 8.1):

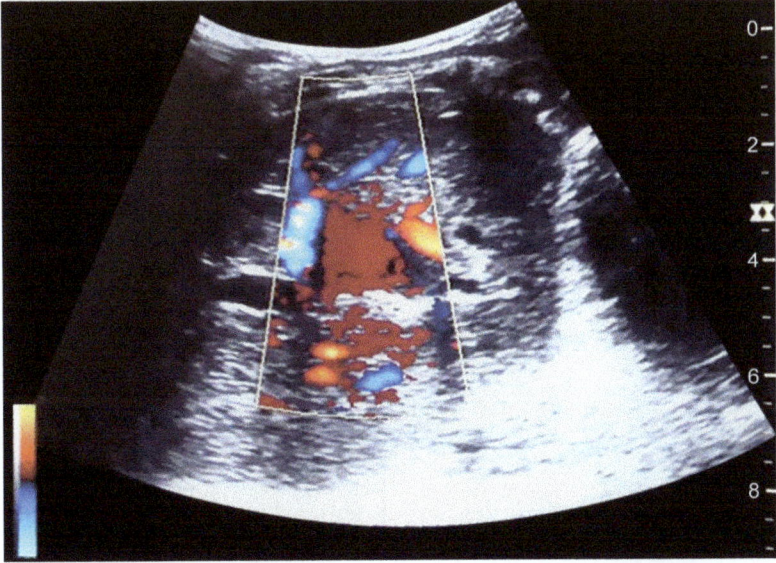

Fig. 8.1: Normal Doppler USG showing good vascularity and flow in segmental vessels.

- The assessment of the renal parenchyma in intrinsic causes of acute kidney injury (AKI).
- Making a differentiation between acute and chronic (AKI vs. CKD).
- Identification of obstructive pathologies and causes.

The B-mode or brightness mode is most often used for renal USG.

Echogenicity is a term, comparing an image as hyperechoic (bright) versus dark (hypoechoic) as compared to standard gray-scale images; an intrinsic property of the quantum of energy absorbed or reflected by the tissues it traverses. The brighter or whiter, something appears and the more echogenic it is. When most of the sound waves are reflected completely as in fat, fibrous tissue and calcified tissues will appear white.

Echogenic nature of the kidney, is a property of the kidneys, as compared to an adjacent solid organ, commonly liver or spleen (providing the liver or spleen are normal) to appear same, bright (hyperechoic) or dark (hypoechoic).

Visualization of the right kidney may be done through the right lobe of the liver, by anterior approach, but the renal lengths viewed from this position may be inaccurate.

The parenchyma of the kidneys is made up of two parts, the cortex and the medulla. Which are usually isoechoic or sometimes hypoechoic.

Both cortex and medulla usually have the same echogenicity, the medulla sometimes appearing darker. Both kidneys usually have same echogenic values.

The dividing line between cortex and medulla is generally identified by the pulsations of the arcuate artery. The medullary fat in the center of the kidney appears hyperechoic when compared to the parenchyma of the kidneys (Fig. 8.2).

The pyramids in the medulla, which hold urine, give a dark appearance located between the cortex and renal sinus.

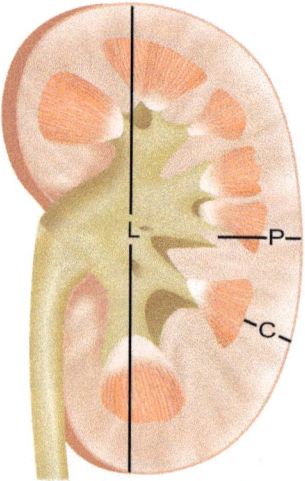

Fig. 8.2: Basic renal anatomy showing cortex (C), medulla, pyramids (P).

Anechoic appearances are produced by all liquid-filled spaces (simple cysts, urine, fresh blood); therefore, blood clots in the urinary space appear echogenic when compared with the renal parenchyma, (acute — hypoechoic, subacute and chronic clots —hyperechogenic).

Traditionally kidneys with parenchyma replaced by fibrous tissue in chronic kidney disease appear more echogenic and however certain acute kidney injury conditions are correlated with raised echogenicity. Inflammatory infiltrates and tissue edema may explain the raised echogenicity (acute interstitial nephritis and glomerulonephritis). Casts with proteinaceous contents composed of Tamm-Horsfall protein and free light chains may be responsible for the hyperechoic appearance of the kidney in acute tubular necrosis (ATN) and myeloma kidney.

Cortical necrosis causes severe usually irreversible AKI and may be suspected by the appearance of a dark, hypoechogenic renal cortex. This may arise from more severe ischemia than ATN as in the hemolytic-uremic syndrome, vasculotoxic snake bite, severe pancreatitis or sepsis, or when all the compensatory mechanisms are working at their maximum limit as in complications of pregnancy, eclampsia or peripartum hemorrhage.

Necrosis of cortical tubular cells, and increased interstitial fluid result in reduced echoic nature of the cortex.

It is important to distinguish cortical necrosis from ATN if possible as it causes only partially reversible AKI at best or is totally irreversible. Ultrasonography however may need to be confirmed with angiography, computerized tomography or in late stages by the presence of calcification on a plain X-ray.

Markedly raised medullary echogenicity, due to highly echogenic calcium deposits and stones, along with a normal looking cortex are pathognomonic of medullary nephrocalcinosis.

Box 8.1 lists the diseases which produce medullary nephrocalcinosis.

An edematous parenchyma may be associated with increased echogenicity, thus diminishing the specificity of bright echotexture for chronic kidney disease, renal appearances suggesting acute kidney injury (Box 8.2).

Although size is usually diminished in chronic kidney disease a few exceptions exist, most notably diabetic kidney disease, multiple myeloma, lymphomatous infiltration renal vein thrombosis, some cases of HIV nephropathy and amyloidosis where size is preserved till late in the disease.

> **Box 1:** Causes of medullary nephrocalcinosis.
> - Medullary sponge kidney
> - Hyperparathyroidism
> - Renal tubular acidosis
> - Hypervitaminosis D
> - Tuberculosis
> - Sarcoidosis
> - Milk-alkali syndrome
> - Sickle cell disease
> - Multiple myeloma
> - Gout
> - Papillary necrosis.

> **Box 2:** Renal appearances suggesting acute kidney injury.
> - Normal or enlarged kidneys
> - Prominent pyramids
> - Increased or decreased echotexture with preserved corticomedullary differentiation.
> - Preservation of parenchymal and cortical thickness at 1.5 and 1 cm respectively.*

*The pulsating arcuate artery marks the boundary between cortex and medulla.

Although kidney sizes should ideally refer to volumes, renal length is most often measured and reported normal kidney length in Indian adults averages 9 cm, depending on body habitus, with a normal range of up to 11 cm; difference of the size of the kidneys in women (left is greater than right by 0.3 cm is observed). Kidneys in women are 0.5 cm smaller than in men. Kidney sizes, less than 8 cm, are usually pathological in individuals less than age 60, reducing lengths are seen after the age of 60. Kidney length also correlates with patient's height weight and body surface area; if these are adjusted for, the normalized kidney sizes for both sexes are similar.

The American College of Radiology (ACR) Appropriateness Criteria (these are a collection of recommendations based on strong evidence, which help the clinician in choosing an imaging modality for a specific clinical condition).

The rating given for ultrasonography in AKI is 9, the highest possible, establishing its merit.

Ultrasound is indicated urgently in cases of AKI, with no identifiable cause, or has risks of obstruction (timeline-within 24 hours).

Within 6 Hours

In cases of suspected pyonephrosis with AKI.

DIAGNOSING AND ASSESSING OBSTRUCTION

Ultrasound is the preferred imaging technique to diagnose obstructive pathologies (1–3% AKI in critical care unit). Clinically significant obstruction (Fig. 8.3), in more than 95% cases, (appears hypoechoic due to retained urine) is seen on ultrasound as dilated urinary collecting system and this is *hydronephrosis* sensitivity is 100% in moderate to severe hydronephrosis. Table 8.1 shows false-positive and false-negative situations (Fig. 8.4 and 8.5).

Use of Color Doppler Ultrasonography

Doppler imaging is used to quantify blood flow and assess its velocity in the vessels of an organ, in this case the kidney. The property of frequency shift of the returning ultrasonographic waves reflected from moving red blood cells is utilized by computers to calculate the velocity. Resistive index (RI) is chosen most frequently to study blood flow because of its reproducibility.

Table 8.1: The false negative and false-positive situations.

False-negatives (obstruction without hydronephrosis)	False-positives (hydronephrosis without obstruction)
Retroperitoneal fibrosis	Pregnancy
Staghorn calculus with obstruction	Vesicoureteric reflux
Dehydration and prerenal AKI	Overdistended bladder
Nonfunctioning obstructed kidney	Megaureter
Very early obstruction	Nephrogenic diabetes insipidus with high flow rates
	Postdeobstruction

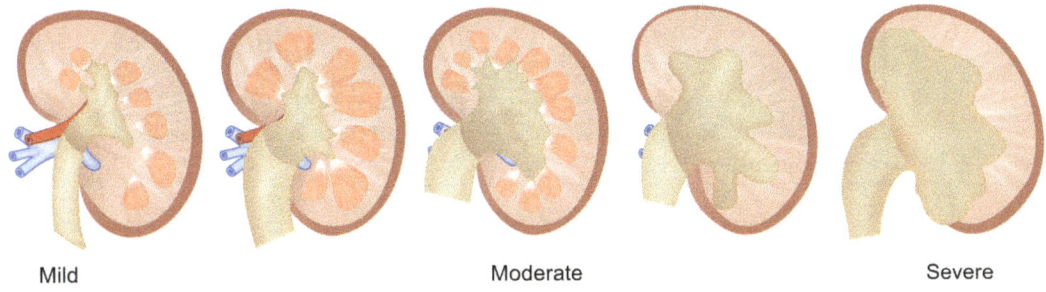

Mild   Moderate   Severe

Fig. 8.3: Grades of hydronephrosis

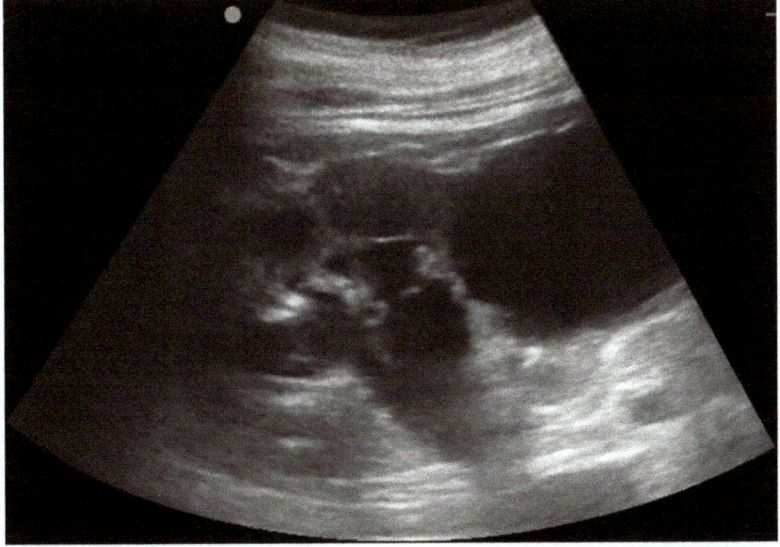

Fig. 8.4: Severe hydronephrosis.

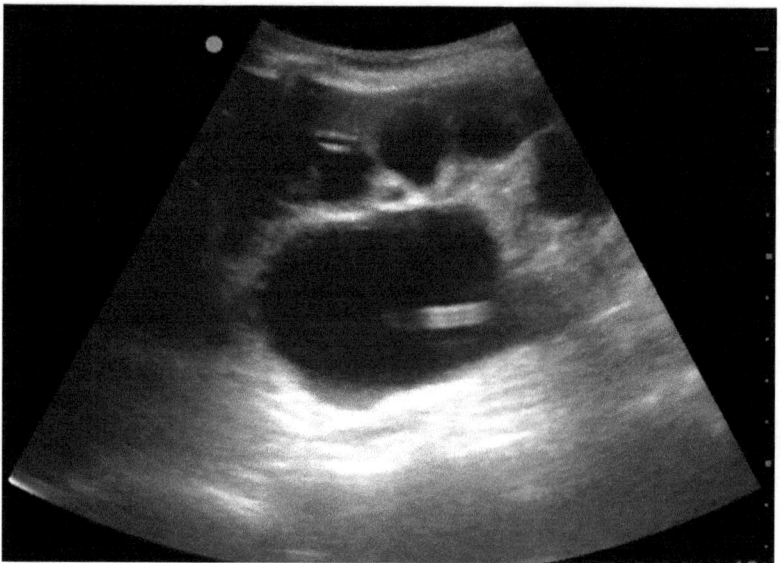

Fig. 8.5: Severe hydronephrosis with stent.

The index is calculated by measuring the blood velocities (systolic and diastolic) from the waveform in the segmental arteries and using the following calculation:

$$RI = \frac{\text{Peak systolic velocity (PSV) - end diastolic velocity (EDV)}}{\text{Peak systolic velocity (PSV)}}$$

Resistive index is indicative of resistance to flow in the intrarenal vessels of the kidney.

Resistive index can be interpretated as follows:

Resistive index ~ 0.6 (0.56–0.66) — normal.

Low—indicates normal renal vascular resistance.

Raised—chronic kidney disease and acute kidney disease, as both parenchymal swelling and fibrosis increase the intrarenal resistance to blood flow and, higher the level of RI, more severe the renal parenchymal damage and worse the outcome.

It is important to know however the limitations of RI measurements, which may be influenced by several independent extrarenal factors, like compliance of blood vessels, systemic vascular resistance (SVR) and heart rates. When the pulse drops (bradycardia), more time is required for flow during diastole to decrease, hence raising the RI, whereas the opposite occurs with increased heart rates, lowering the RI. Additionally, cases having extensive arterial narrowing, caused by diffuse atherosclerosis or reduced vascular compliance, a consequence of vascular stiffening, in old patients, may cause a raised RI, even in the absence of renal dysfunction.

Importantly in suspected obstruction the increase in RI may precede the development of dilatation of the collecting system and returns to normal after deobstruction (Box 8.3).

Box 8.3: Use of resistive index in ICU—acute kidney injury.

Increased RI
- ATN
- Obstruction
- Hepatorenal syndrome
- Acute rejection following transplant
- Predicting development of AKI in septic shock, cardiopulmonary bypass and trauma
- Assessing degree or severity of AKI

Normal RI
Prerenal azotemia
Glomerulonephritis
Predicting recovery from AKI

(RI: Resistive index; ICU: Intensive care unit; AKI: Acute kidney injury; ATN: Acute tubular necrosis)

Use of Ultrasonography in the Early Post-transplant Period

It may be applied for diagnostic and monitoring purposes from very early on, in the post-transplant period, or even intraoperatively establishing thus establishing baseline parameters for follow-up scanning, besides evaluation of the causes of early graft dysfunction, it can be also utilized for interventions like real time guided renal biopsy and drainage of fluid collection.

An initial evaluation is usually done even in normally functioning allograft in the first 24–48 hours post-transplantation. Evaluation for kidney sizes, echoic nature, study of collecting system and ureters and for any obvious collections that may develop after the surgery. Doppler imaging (PW/CW) is used to assess renal and iliac arteries or blood vessels as well as intrarenal vessels. Flow quantification is then done by calculating the RI, PI and ratio of systole to diastole.

An allograft kidney has a similar ultrasound appearance to the native one; but is located more superficially, and thus higher frequency transducers can be utilized. A slight increase in size is observed during the first-few weeks, reaching till 32% of the starting length till the 4th week. Collecting system of an adequately functioning transplant is often slightly dilated, possibly due to a large volume of urine produced and a degree of vesicoureteric reflux despite the antireflux measures taken at surgery and loss of the ureter's tonicity from denervation.

In an unobstructed allograft, only minimal dilatation, restricted to the renal pelvis is noted, while dilatation in infundibula or the calyces could point towards outflow obstruction (significant).

Blood flow in healthy kidneys post-transplant are seen better than those of the native kidney, with color flow is expected to reach the renal capsule and segmental, interlobar blood having RI is less than or equal to 0.8 by spectral Doppler.

Common causes of acute allograft dysfunction include:
- Acute tubular necrosis
- Acute rejection
- Acute calcineurin inhibitor toxicity
- Infection

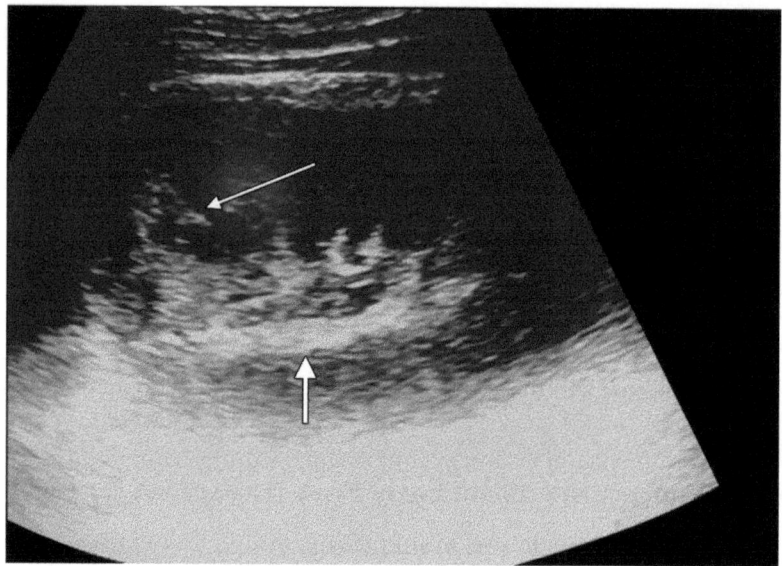

Fig. 8.6: Emphysematous pyelonephritis with gas in the pelvis and renal parenchyma (arrows).

The ultrasonographic appearances of all these conditions are nonspecific with allograft swelling prominent pyramids, and absent or reversal of end-diastolic flow in allograft kidney.

In a specific infection, the immunosuppressed recipient is prone to specific infections, like emphysematous pyelonephritis, in which gas forming organisms ferment glucose to produce gas which is visualized as a hyperechoic shadow in either the pelvicalyceal system or the renal parenchyma. Although CT scan is the gold standard for diagnosing and staging emphysematous pyelonephritis, in very unstable patient's bedside ultrasonography can provide the diagnosis and also allow percutaneous drainage which may be lifesaving (Fig. 8.6).

Air within the renal allograft substance produces a bright hyperechoic line with reverberation artifacts seen distally, while focal rounded, weakly shadowing and echogenic structures within the collecting system are seen commonly with fungus balls. It is another major complication in allograft kidneys especially in patients with new onset diabetes after transplantation.

The greatest role of the duplex USG in allograft kidneys is in vascular events which may be catastrophic, arterial and venous thrombosis. Arterial thrombosis of the main renal artery or the iliac artery is characterized by sudden absence of vascularity and flow in the allograft. In some cases a demarcation of flow may be visible between the iliac and the renal artery or the presence of an echogenic thrombus at the anastomotic site may be visible however these are late signs. A segmental infarct produces a focal, hypoechoic, typically wedge-shaped area with perfusion defects on color Doppler.

In venous thrombosis, absent or reversal of diastolic flow in main or intrarenal arteries with absent flow or an echogenic thrombus in the renal vein may be the first sign followed by systolic, thrombectomy may salvage the graft if an early diagnosis is made.

URINE LEAKS, URINOMAS AND LYMPHOCELES

An anechoic fluid collection with clearly seen borders, no internal echoes or septations are seen with urine leaks and urinomas. The collection may sometimes rapidly increase in size necessitating drainage, accurately done under ultrasound guidance. A urine leak or seroma or lymphocele is diagnosed by higher creatinine level in the liquid compared to the same serum levels. Urinoma abscesses can follow if undiagnosed. Minor leaks can be attended to by nephrostomies, done percutaneously or stent insertion, again under ultrasound guidance.

Raised creatinine, because of obstruction (hydronephrosis) can also be easily picked up, however the examination should always be performed after asking the patient to void and with an empty bladder in contrast to native kidneys. This is because a mild degree of hydronephrosis is always seen when the bladder is full caused by the small degree of reflux. Internal echoes in the collecting system suggest pyonephrosis, fungal infections, clots, or tumor. Lymphoceles, hematomas, abscesses, and urinomas may cause external ureteral compression with resulting hydronephrosis.

INTERVENTIONS USING ULTRASONOGRAPHIC GUIDANCE

Few major interventions may be carried out using portable bedside USG in critically-ill patients on both native and allograft kidneys.
1. Percutaneous renal biopsy (Fig. 8.7)
2. Percutaneous nephrostomy
3. Drainage of perigraft fluid collection in allograft kidneys.

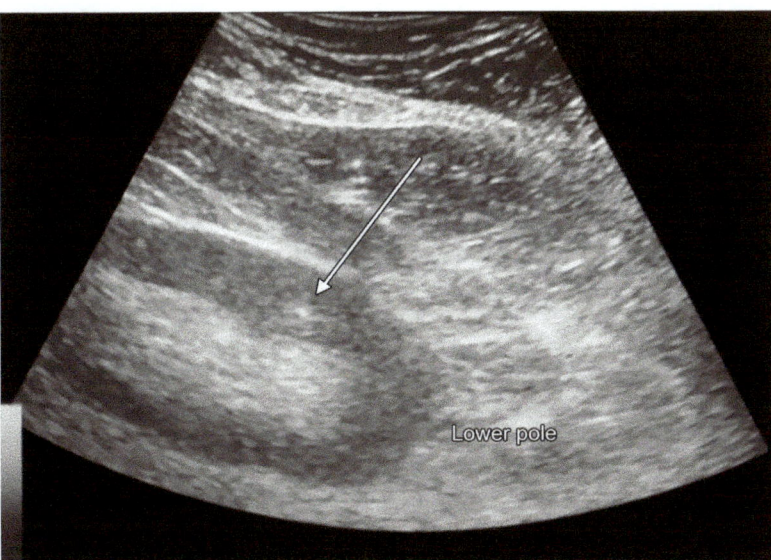

Fig. 8.7: Ultrasonography guided native kidney percutaneous kidney biopsy. The biopsy needle tip seen as white dot (arrow).

FURTHER READING

1. Cosgrove DO, Chan KE. Renal transplants: what ultrasound can and cannot do. Ultrasound Q. 2008;24(2):77-87.
2. Faubel S, Patel NU, Lockhart ME, et al. Renal relevant radiology: use of ultrasonography in patients with AKI. Clin J Am Soc Nephrol. 2014;9(2):382-94.
3. Kolofousi C, Stefanidis K, Cokkinos DD, et al. Ultrasonographic features of kidney transplants and their complications: an imaging review. ISRN Radiology. 2013:1-12.
4. Martino P, Galosi AB. Atlas of Ultrasonography in Urology, Andrology, and Nephrology, 1st edition. Philadelphia: Springer; 2017.
5. National Clinical Guideline Centre. Acute kidney injury: prevention, detection and management up to the point of renal replacement therapy (Clinical Guidelines, No. 169). London: NICE; 2013.

CHAPTER 9

Role of Ultrasound in the Liver Transplant Patient

Manish Pathak

INTRODUCTION

Uses of ultrasound in the perioperative phase in real time are invaluable tools for the surgeon.

The findings, many times can change the planned approaches and hence benefit the patient.

Liver ultrasound in the perioperative phase is useful in staging of malignancies, providing help during metastasectomy, procedures with malignancies like ablations, checking patency and flow within vessels, biliary pathology identification, and as a guide during liver transplant surgeries.

It is advisable to use a specific probe and method to do such examinations for best benefits to the patients.

EQUIPMENT

Transducer Requirements

Special probes, like a 5 MHz type or a curvilinear probe are commonly used with available pule wave and color Doppler facilities.

We should be able to obtain good resolution of images in the objects of interest both in near and far fields.

Probe Asepsis

- Various methods are in use, some indigenous and some slightly expensive.
- Some methods being used include sterile glove drains (condom like sheaths) and custom made probe sheaths (mainly for perioperative probes)
- For proper sterility to be maintained, the sheath should cover nearly the entire length of the probe and its attached cord (more than 1 m).
- Artifacts are seen as disturbing images if the tight fit is not made.
- Appropriate care should be taken to avoid sharp objects near such "sterile" probes as it could potentially lead to a contamination situation.

Use of Ultrasound in the Liver Transplant Patient

Proper identification of patent vessels and also seeing the integrity of anastomosed vessels may be desired.

Sometimes, when disparity occurs between the recipient and donor vessel sizes, grafts are used to bypass or "bridge" the defect, the patency of which can be well confirmed by ultrasound.

Ultrasound is useful also to identify vascular injuries that may occur in the intraoperative period, (like hepatic artery).

The use can extend to even identify relatively avascular planes which may then be utilized for procedures like location of right lobe during split liver transplants harvests.

This site is usually seen around 1–2 cm near the hepatic vein (to its right).

Ultrasound may identify any accessory hepatic veins, which may require separate procedures for joining, in addition to localizing the hepatic veins which drain the fifth and eighth liver segments.

Complications related to transplants like thrombus formation and extension, left back vascular structures (vena cava) are also detected quite accurately by the ultrasound use.

Use of Ultrasound in the Intraoperative Phase

Pathologies of the liver like tumors and its differentiation into solid, cystic or varied are detected much more accurately when compared to conventional methods like transabdominal ultrasound or even scans.

The ability to localize pathologies located close to vascular structures helps in more safe resections of the liver tissue.

Colorectal cancers are evaluated more thoroughly, better staging is possible, in addition to giving valuable information on the baseline liver disease.

Thus, it is reasonably quite sensitive (98%) and specific (95%) for the metastases detection (colorectal) (Schmidt group).

CONCLUSION

Ultrasound done during the perioperative phase can give crucial and sometimes lifesaving information to the surgeon.

This translates into better, more accurate and tailor made care, and safety during the procedure.

The clinical outcome of such patients has shown a good trend.

With the field of transplants taking off in our country, the future is likely to be crowded by more and more extended uses of the point of care ultrasound!

13
CHAPTER

Ultrasound-guided Nerve Blocks: Basics

Vrushali Ponde

"The secret of joy in work is contained in one word—excellence. To know how to do something well is to enjoy it."—Pearl S Buck

INTRODUCTION

Regional anesthesiology is one of the most fascinating aspects of anesthesiology. It is the best tool we have to handle perioperative pain with no side effects of other systemic analgesics. A perioperative experience of minimal pain is always a goal of a committed anesthesiologist and regional anesthesia, used skill fully, is one most efficient ways of handling it. Nerve block is a part of regional anesthesia and by itself can have complication and failures. Intravascular injections, intraneural injections and failures of the nerve blocks are the most discouraging issues. Ultrasound guidance had changed this by adding a new dimension of real-time visualization of nerves to be blocked, the insertion and placement of needle right next the nerve of interest and finally injection of the local anesthetic around the nerve. It is logically appealing to expect that the rate of complication should decrease and the success rate of nerve blocks should increase. This has also been shown by clinical evidence.

BASIC PRINCIPLES

Few basic principles are given here to follow.

Nerve Identification

Nerve identification is the very basis of all regional blocks.

Scanning of the nerves is done either in transverse sections (Fig. 13.1) or longitudinal. It is best to scan nerves in transverse section for block procedures because transverse scans are easier to work in, than longitudinal scans. In transverse section, the nerves cast a typical circular to oval "honeycomb"-like appearance. The "honeycomb" appearance of the nerve is due to the fascicles cut in transverse section, which appear like hypoechoic images with

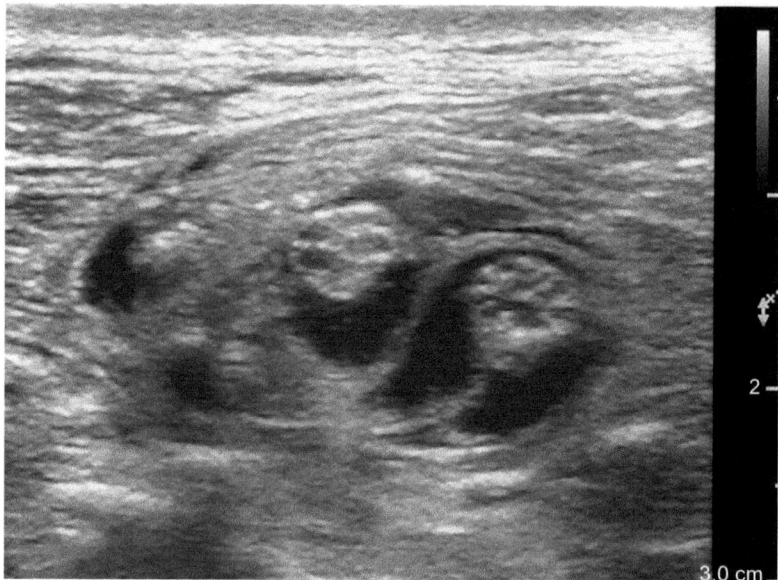

Fig. 13.1: Transverse section of tibial and common peroneal nerve surrounded by local anesthetic solution.

the intervening hyperechoic tissue. The perineurium surrounding the fascicles imparts a hyperechoic interface (hyperechoic rim). The classical example is the sciatic nerve. It could be worthwhile to trace the nerve along its course to identify the path and differentiate it from the adjacent tendons, which disappear in the muscle mass when traced proximally.

Although all nerves are hyperechoic, the nerves in the neck and the axilla are hypoechoic with a hyperechoic rim (e.g. brachial plexus interscalene) and these nerves commonly run together with vascular structure. Therefore, it is important to distinguish small vessels, which also have a similar appearance, from small monofascicular nerves. Visible pulsation and color flow mapping can easily differentiate them.

Equipment

Ultrasound machine with high-frequency linear (HFL) probe is suitable for most peripheral nerves. Although deeper nerves can be better seen by curvilinear low-frequency probes. Hockey stick probe (SLA) is convenient for pediatric imaging due to its smaller footprint size. However, HFL probe is also used in children with comfort in certain blocks such as sciatic, lumbar plexus, femoral and axillary blocks. For neck blocks in very small babies [interscalene, internal jugular vein (IJV) cannulation], hockey stick probe (SLA) is more suitable.

Needle and Probe Relationship

"In-Plane" Approach

In this approach, the needle is put in a direction parallel to the plane of the ultrasound beam. The entire needle shaft and tip is visualized approaching the target with this technique.

"Out-of-Plane" Approach

The path of insertion of the needle crosses the plane of the ultrasound beam. The full needle including the tip is not seen by this method. The needle tip in transverse section is visualized moving toward the chosen target.

In the next section, we shall discuss few most commonly ultrasound-guided nerve blocks in every day work.

UPPER EXTREMITY BLOCKS

Since the vascular structures and nerves occur together in this region (brachial plexus), we use the vascular structures as landmark for the nerve identification.

The choice and approach are many and would depend on where the intervention is being done.

Brachial plexus area is unique in its composition.

INTERSCALENE BLOCK

Indications

Surgeries involving the lateral two-thirds of the clavicle, shoulder, proximal humerus as well as the shoulder joint.

Applied Anatomy

Brachial plexus divides into superior, middle, inferior trunks which then descend in the interscalene groove (located between scalenus anterior and scalenus medius). They lie as an oblique stack of dark rings in this space.

Block Procedure

Supine position with neck turned to opposite side.
- The probe is held in the posterior triangle of the neck, in a transverse way.
- The location is at or just below the cricoid cartilage.
- Note the marker on probe, facing laterally.

Ultrasound Scan

Anteriorly, visualize the sternocleidomastoid muscle. Scalene muscles (anterior and middle) are seen laterally (Fig. 13.2). Identify nerve trunks between the two muscles. The subclavian artery and the brachial plexus, which surrounds the vessel can be located by inferior angulation toward the base of the neck, above the clavicle scanning.

Probe and Needle Relationship

Insert the needle in plane with the ultrasound beam, or even from a position lateral to the probe. The nerve trunks, being superficial in this area cause good visualization of the needle

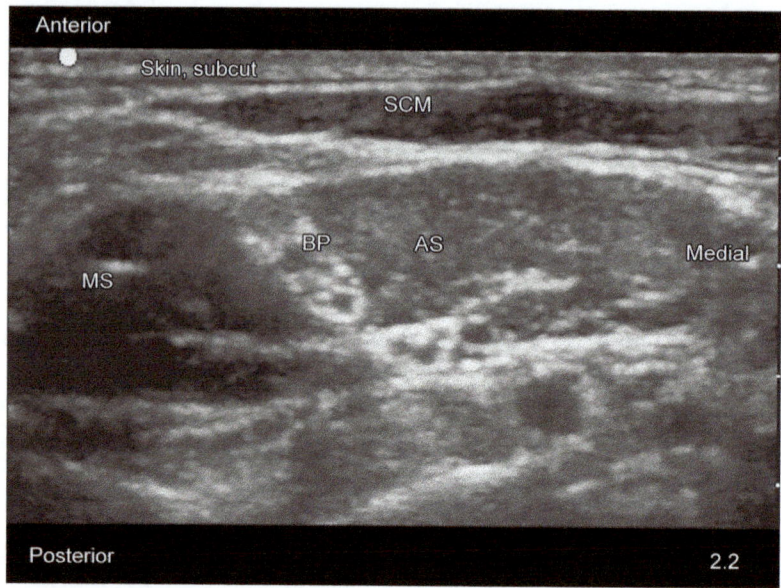

Fig. 13.2: Interscalene approach brachial plexus block.
(SCM: sternocleidomastoid; BP: brachial plexus; MS: medial scalene; AS: anterior scalene)

tip and shaft. This is followed by lodging the tip in between any two of the trunks (interscalene groove). The local anesthetic is then injected.

BRACHIAL PLEXUS BLOCK (SUPRACLAVICULAR APPROACH)

The brachial plexus (trunks), divides at this region, which can be well located and nerve block given under ultrasound guidance.

Indications

All procedures below and at elbow region (hand and forearm included).

Applied Anatomy

Brachial plexus has upper (C5, C6), middle (C7), lower (C8-T12) trunks in this area.

The artery (subclavian) is located in a position which is anterior and medial to the plexus in the interscalene triangle.

Procedure for Nerve Block

Supine position with neck turned to opposite side.
The probe is held in the supraclavicular fossa of the neck, in a transverse way.
Note the marker on probe, facing laterally.

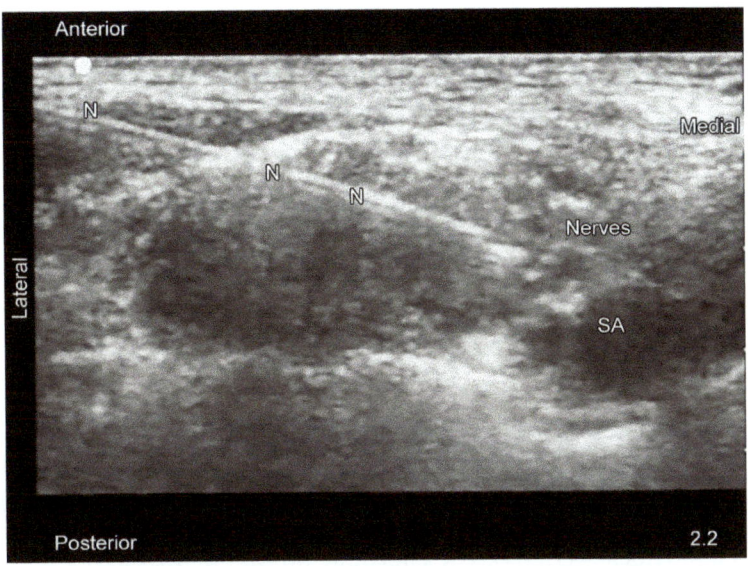

Fig. 13.3: Subclavian perivascular or supraclavicular approach brachial plexus block. (N: needle; SA: subclavian artery)

Ultrasound Findings

We look for a "bunch of grapes" appearance, dark ring-like structures which are hypoechoic located in a direction which is superior and lateral to the subclavian artery (seen as a structure pulsating above the 1st rib).

Please refer to the diagram for a transverse section of this anatomy (Fig. 13.3).

Needle and Probe Relationship

An "in-plane" approach is used.

The movement of the needle is from lateral to medial, point of insertion being just near the lateral aspect of the probe.

Locate the tip of the needle just near the nerve, and deliver the injection/local anesthetic.

BRACHIAL PLEXUS BLOCK (INFRACLAVICULAR APPROACH)

The brachial plexus is blocked at the level of the cords with this approach.

Indications

Ideal for forearm and hand procedures.

Applied Anatomy

The cords which run along the subclavian artery and/or axillary artery are situated in the infraclavicular fossa.

The neurovascular bundle is located posterior to the pectoralis major and minor muscles. The ribs and pleura are seen in a direction medial to the bundle.

Procedure for Nerve Block

Supine Position

With the arm to be blocked alongside the subject.

The infraclavicular area is scanned in the parasagittal plane below the coracoid process in children, with the orientation marker of the probe toward the clavicle.

Ultrasound Findings

In the parasagittal section at the level of infraclavicular region (Fig. 13.4), the scan shows the pectoralis major and minor muscles, and subclavian artery with subclavian vein. The cords are also seen. The cords appear as hyperechoic structures surrounding the subclavian artery.

We can identify the cord (lateral) in a location anterior to the artery.

The posterior cord is seen posterior to the artery. It is difficult to see the medial cord. The medial cord is situated in between the artery and the vein.

Needle and Probe Relationship

An "in-plane" approach is used.

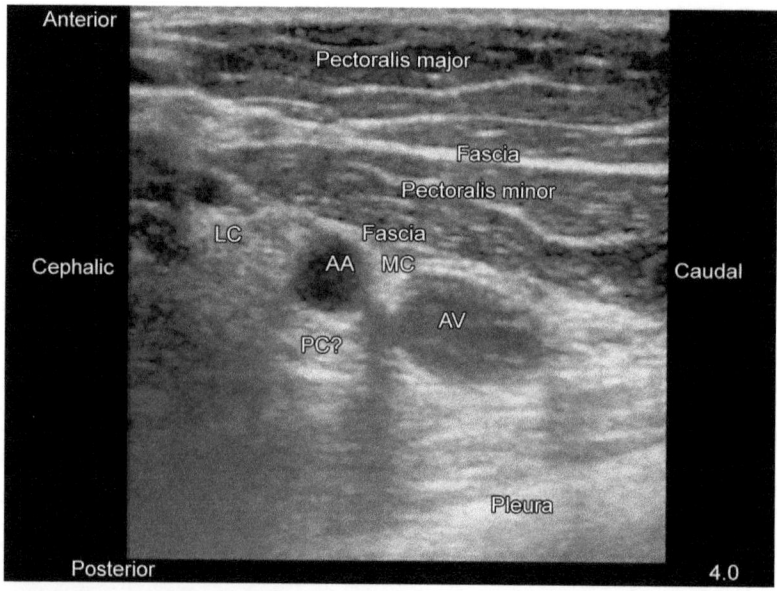

Fig. 13.4: Infraclavicular approach brachial plexus block.
(LC: lateral cord; MC: medial cord; PC: posterior cord; AA: axillary artery; AV: axillary vein)

The needle is advanced at an angle of around 40–60° with the skin, from the cephalad area of the probe, in the long axis of the probe. Advancement of tip is observed in real-time image to target the posterior cord (the needle tip has to be lodged on the posterior aspect of the artery). Local anesthetic spread posterior to the artery or a periarterial U-shaped spread is accepted.

BRACHIAL PLEXUS BLOCK (AXILLARY LEVEL)

The terminal branches are approached with this approach.

Indications

This block is for hand and forearm surgeries.

Applied Anatomy

The lateral, medial and posterior cords give terminal branches namely median, ulnar, radial, musculocutaneous and axillary nerves.

The axillary and musculocutaneous nerves are usually spared with this approach because they leave the plexus at the level of coracoid process. Axillary artery in the axilla is accompanied by these nerves (median, ulnar and radial nerve) and is blocked by the axillary approach.

Nerve block involving the musculocutaneous nerve may be attempted separately.

Block Procedure

Supine Position

The target arm is abducted to form a 90° angle with the trunk (body).

The arm is rotated externally and bent at the elbow.

The footprint is placed transversely in the axilla, in a direction parallel to the trunk and perpendicular to the arm with the orientation marker toward the head of the patient. The probe can be moved distally to visualize the musculocutaneous nerve.

Ultrasound Findings (Figs. 13.5 and 13.6)

The ultrasound scan shows a pulsatile axillary artery.

A compressible structure (axillary vein) is located just near the axillary artery.

The median, radial and ulnar nerves are located around the artery.

Median is situated anterior to the axillary artery (12 o'clock). The ulnar nerve is located in a direction medial to the axillary artery and axillary vein (2 o'clock), it lies between two vascular structures (Figs. 13.5 and 13.7).

Radial nerve is found in a direction behind the artery (6 o'clock).

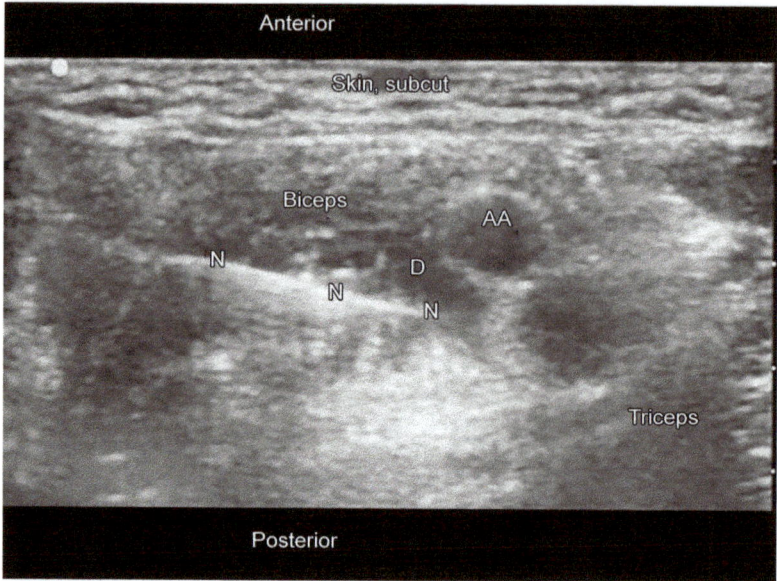

Figs. 13.5: Axillary approach to brachial plexus.
(AA: axillary artery; N: needle; D: drug)

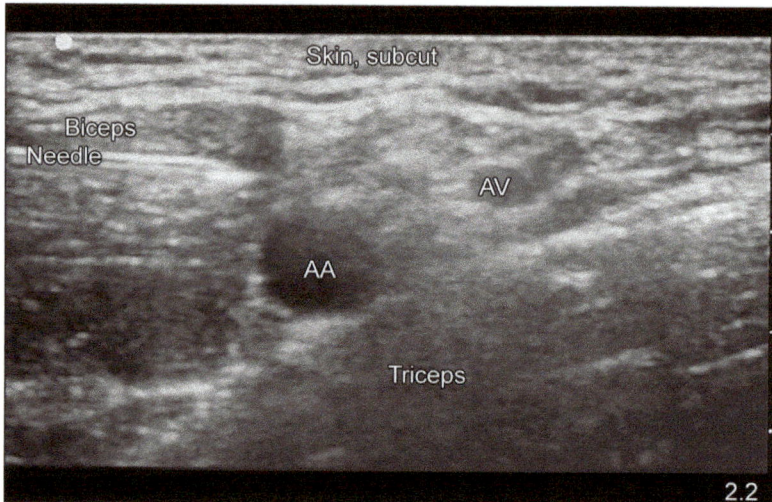

Fig 13.6: Axillary approach to brachial plexus. Needle directed towards the median nerve location.
(AA: axillary artery; AV: axillary vein)

MUSCULOCUTANEOUS NERVE BLOCK

The probe is moved a bit distally to visualize the nerve.

The biceps and coracobrachialis muscles are seen, and the nerve lies in between the two muscles.

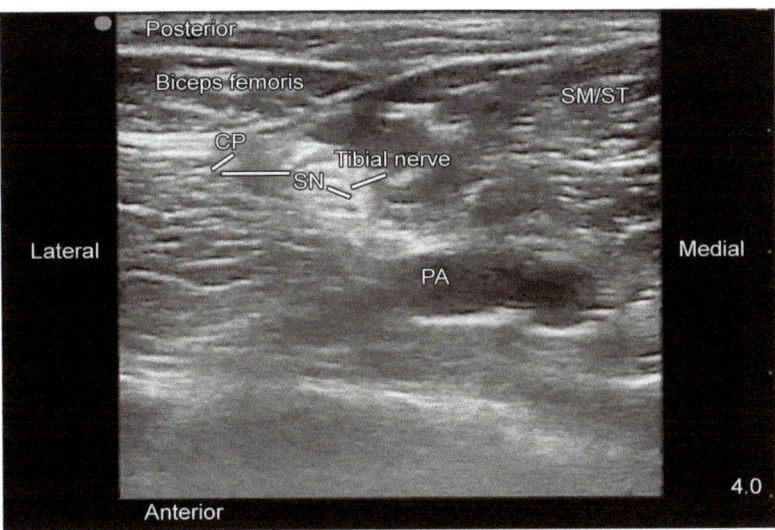

Fig. 13.7: Popliteal sciatic nerve.
(SM/ST: semimembranosus, semitendinosus; PA: popliteal artery; CP: common peroneal, SN: sciatic nerve)

Using the "in-plane" approach is advisable, and the needle-probe relationship is similar to axillary block.

LOWER LIMB BLOCKS

Using sciatic and femoral blocks, adequate anesthesia can be imparted for lower limb surgeries.

A dual nerve supply to lower limbs (from branches of lumbar and sacral plexus) necessitates a dual block in this area.

This is unlike the upper limb.

SCIATIC NERVE BLOCK

Indications

Surgeries below the knee, calf, ankle and foot can be performed under sciatic block (with a supplemental femoral/saphenous nerve block).

Sciatic Nerve and its Course in the Thigh

The largest peripheral nerve in the body, the sciatic nerve, from the sacral plexus, arises from the ventral rami of L4 to S3.

It consists of two different nerves, the common peroneal and the tibial, both enclosed in an epineural sheath.

The sciatic nerve exits from the pelvis via the greater sciatic foramen, travels deep to the gluteus maximus muscle, in between the greater trochanter and ischial tuberosity, to enter the thigh.

In the proximal thigh, it is surrounded by the adductor magnus and long head of biceps femoris, and descends in the groove between biceps femoris muscle laterally, and semimembranosus muscle and semitendinosus muscle medially. At a variable distance proximal to the popliteal fossa, it ends in common peroneal and tibial nerves.

SCIATIC NERVE BLOCK (POPLITEAL AREA)

Applied Anatomy

In the region of the posterior part of thigh, we find the common peroneal and tibial nerves (branches of sciatic). The best way to deliver the "block" will be to directly see the branching of the nerve, and inject under direct vision. The nerve in the popliteal fossa is seen in close proximity with the semimembranous (posterior and lateral) and semitendinosus (posterior and medial) muscles.

Indications

Better for foot and ankle surgeries.

Position of the Patient

Lateral or supine with leg flexed at hip and knee, and elevation of the limb, to give place to maneuver the probe in the fossa.

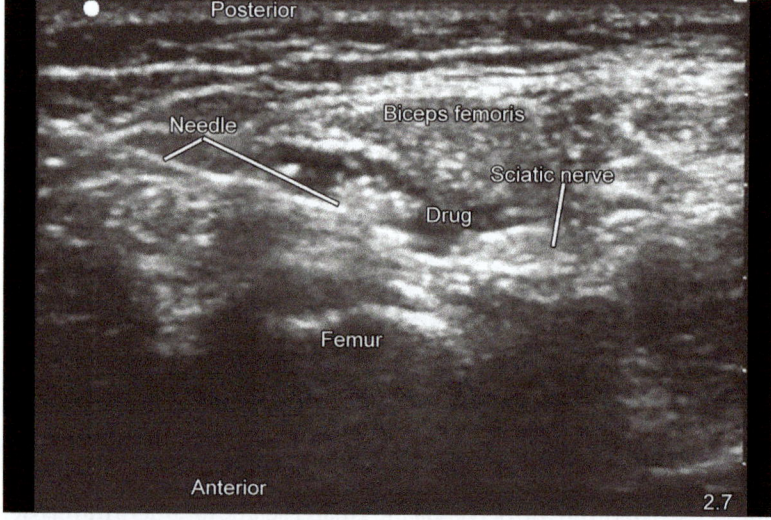

Fig 13.8: Transverse scan at the infragluteal level.

Procedure

The popliteal crease is located, and we go 5–7 cm proximal to this crease.

The probe is placed in a direction perpendicular to the long axis of the limb, with the marker of orientation facing laterally. Moving from lateral to medial side the sciatic nerve is approached by the needle.

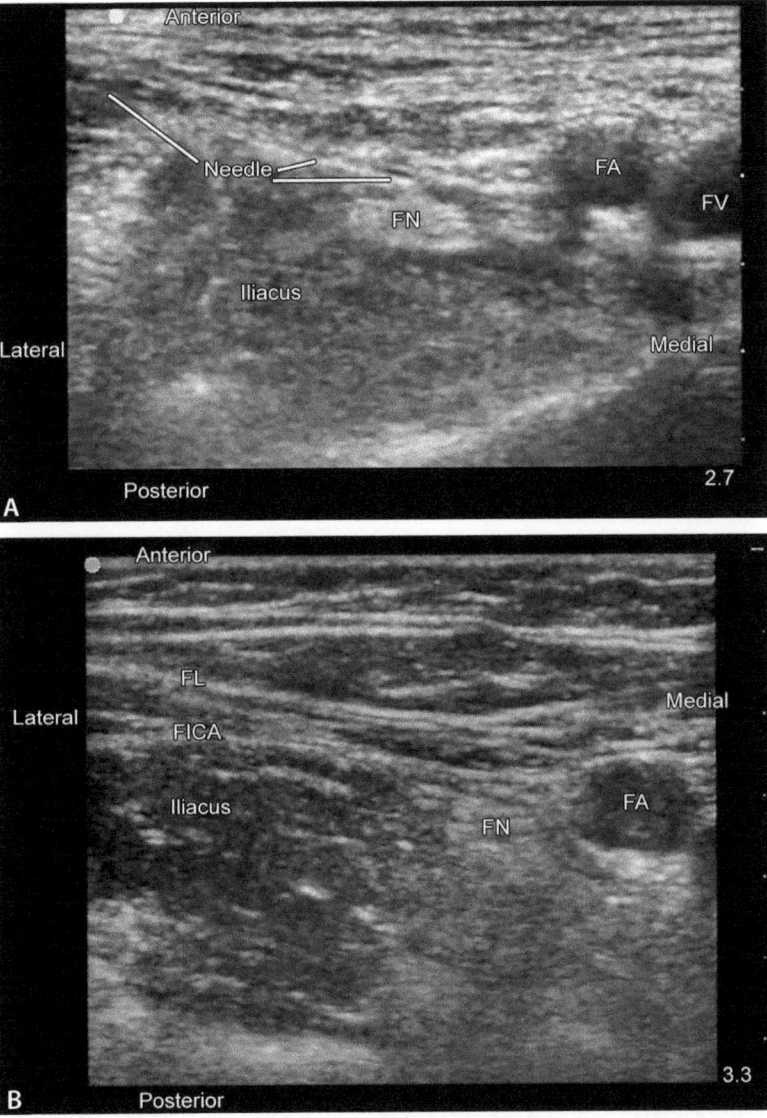

Fig. 13.10: Transverse scan at the level of inguinal crease showing femoral nerve and related structures. (FN: femoral nerve; FA: femoral artery; FL: fascia lata; FV: femoral vein; FICA: fascia iliaca compartment analgesia)

Ultrasound Findings

We look for a round/oval hyperechoic structure with a pattern-like fascicle.

This is done in transverse direction (Fig. 13.8). The sciatic nerve is seen posterior and lateral to the popliteal artery and vein.

The nerve is surrounded by the following structures posteromedially-semimembranosus and semitendinosus, and posterolaterally biceps femoris.

SCIATIC NERVE BLOCK (INFRAGLUTEAL APPROACH)

Applied Anatomy

In infragluteal region, the nerve lies posterior to adductor magnus. The gluteus maximus lies posterolateral to the sciatic nerve, the biceps femoris lies on the posterior and medial aspect.

We identify the gluteus maximus and biceps femoris muscle located from posterior to anterior. It is located anterior to biceps femoris muscle and gluteus maximus. The nerve is seen as a flattened/elliptical/oval structure, when you see the femur in the anterior part of the image. Then identify the posterior cutaneous nerve (Fig. 13.9A).

Under real-time guidance, the needle tip is positioned near the nerve and injections are given. Confirmation of proper injection technique is done if we see a dark hypoechoic shadow produced by the injection increasing in size (due to drug spread). The nerve is seen as getting pushed away from this shadow.

FEMORAL NERVE BLOCK

Applied Anatomy

The femoral nerve arises from the lumbar plexus and it arises from L2 to L5. At the level of femoral crease, the femoral artery is medial, and iliopsoas muscle posterior. The profunda femoris artery and superficial femoral artery are the two branches formed by the femoral artery and are seen during ultrasound imaging.

Block Procedure

Supine position, with the target leg in slight external rotation. Probe is placed parallel along the inguinal crease, with orientation marker facing laterally.

The insertion point is immediately lateral to the probe. The needle is visualized as it moves medially toward the probe. The tip is placed, under direct vision anterior or posterior to the nerve, and injection is given (Fig. 13.9B).

Profunda femoris artery is seen deeper to the femoral artery. In such cases, the scan should be followed proximally toward the inguinal ligament by moving the probe toward the inguinal ligament to visualize main femoral artery. The calculated amount of drug is put adjacent to the nerve.

Note: This write up gives only a glimpse of what is possible with ultrasound application to regional anesthesia.

In conclusion, real-time objective nerve blocks are possible with this technology. It is here to stay and has changed the entire perspective toward nerve blocks.

FURTHER READING

1. Antonakakis J, Ting P, Sites B. Ultrasound-guided regional anesthesia for peripheral nerve blocks: an evidence-based outcome review. Anaesthesiol Clin. 2011:29(2);179-91.
2. Davis JJ. Atlas of ultrasound-guided regional anesthesia. Anesthesiology 2011: 114: 471.
3. Nix CM, Margarido CB, Awad IT, et al. A scoping review of the evidence for teaching ultrasound-guided regional anesthesia regional. Anesth Pain Med. 2013:38(6); 471–80.
4. Ponde V. An illustrative manual of ultrasound guided regional anesthesia for children & adults Mumbai Bhalani publication; 3rd edn. 2019.
5. Wahal C, Kumar A, Pyati S. Advances in regional anaesthesia: A review of current practice, newer techniques and outcomes. Indian J Anaesth [serial online] 2018 [cited 2019 Jun 13];62:94-102.

Index

Page numbers followed by *b* refer to box, *f* refer to figure, and *t* refer to table.

A

Abdominal aorta 84*f*
  normal appearance of 84*f*
  scanning of 83
Abdominal aortic
  aneurysm 83, 84*f*
    ruptured 83
    diameter 83
    dissection 85
Abdominal trauma, penetrating 143
Abdominal wall hematomas 190
Abscesses 113
Absorption 9
Acalculous cholecystitis 96
Accidental esophageal intubation 26
Accurate puncture, rate of 192
Acoustic
  impedance 8
  shadowing 17*f*
Adductor magnus 186
Advanced trauma life support 140
Aeration loss
  moderate 45
  severe 45
Air 31, 96
  bronchogram 37*f*
  mucosal interface 22, 23*f*, 24*f*
Airway 141
  assessment, probe orientation for 21*f*
  for emergencies, ultrasound of 20
Akinesia 72
Allen test 165, 166
  modified 166
Allograft kidney 112, 113
Allograft swelling prominent pyramids 112
American College of Radiology 108
Anesthesiologist anesthesia 175
Anesthesiology, fascinating aspects of 175
Anesthetists 141
Aorta 71, 98
  and stroke volume, velocity-time integral of 55
  long-axis of 84*f*
  longitudinal section of 85*f*

Aortic regurgitation 71, 71*f*
  Doppler assessment of 71*f*
Aortic sonography, limitations of 85
Aortic stenosis 69-71
Aortic valve 49
Apical four-chamber view 49, 50*f*
Apical five-chamber view 49, 51*f*
Artefact, mirror image 19*f*
Arterial cannulation 173
Arterial margins 166
Artery 130, 164, 166, 167*f*
  commonly accessed 165
Arytenoid cartilage 22
Ascites, cause of new-onset 190
Aspiration 188
Atrial contraction 74
Axial resolution 10, 10*f*
Axillary
  artery 165, 179-182
  nerves 181
  vein 180-182

B

B-mode 11, 12*f*
Barcode sign 39*f*
Basilic vein 161, 163
Beads, string of 23
Bedside lung ultrasound in emergency 31, 46, 47
Bent-knee appearance 68, 69*f*
Biceps femoris muscle 184, 186
Bilateral lung fields 35
Biliary pathology identification 115
Bladder perforation 190
Block procedure 177
Blood 5
  clots 107
  vessel
    compliance of 110
    diameter 132
BLUE protocol 47*f*
Blunt abdominal trauma 142
Blunt trauma 144

Body of pancreas 98
Bone 5, 156
Bony structures, appearance of 157f
Bowel
    gas 85
    obstruction 104
    perforation 190
    ultrasound of 93, 102
    wall, thickness of 102
    with contents, dilated 104
Brachial artery 165
Brachial plexus 177-179, 182f
    block 178, 179, 179f, 181
        interscalene approach 178f
    interscalene 176
Brachiocephalic vein 163
Brain death 118, 135
Brain injuries, severe 118
Brainstem reflexes, assessing for 117
Breathing 142
Bronchial tube placement, double lumen 25
Bronchoscopic guidance 194
Bulky pancreas 100f
Bull's eye 168, 170f

C

Calcineurin inhibitor toxicity, acute 111
Cardiac interventional procedures 189
Cardiac output, measurement of 62
Cardiac probe 189
Cardiac tamponade 57
Cardiac trauma 144
Cardiac ultrasound, focused 49, 72
Cardiac valves, focused assessment of 65
Cardiopulmonary bypass 111
Carotid artery 165f
    external 126, 127
    internal 126, 127
    plaque in 126f
Catheter placement 173
Cellular relengthening rates 74
Central nervous
    catheter 173
    system 137
Cephalic vein 162
Cerebral artery
    anterior 127, 131f
    middle 127, 129f, 133f
    posterior 128
Cerebral circulatory arrest 133f, 135, 135f
Cerebrovascular disease, extracranial 125
Cervical, trauma visualization of 137
Chest trauma 145

Cholecystitis 93
Choledocholithiasis 93
Cholelithiasis 93
Circle of Willis 129f
    part of 128f
Clavicle 177
Clots 113
Collapsibility index 60
Collapsibility, loss of 89f
Color Doppler 166
    ultrasonography 108
Color flow 72f
    imaging 13, 14
    mapping 66, 68f
Comet-tail artifact 15, 16f, 21
Common bile duct 93, 96-98, 101
Common carotid artery 126, 127, 163
Common femoral
    artery 89, 164
    vein 89
Communicating artery
    anterior 127
    posterior 128
Compression test 88
    normal 89f
Computed tomography 83
Constricted pupil 121f
Contralateral temporal bone 129f
Coracobrachialis muscles 182
Cord, posterior 180
Cornea 118
Cortex, echoic nature of 107
Cortical tubular cells, necrosis of 107
Cost-effective imaging tool 188
Cranial nerves 117
Cricoid cartilage 20, 24
    transverse view of 23f
Cricothyroid membrane 20, 24
Cricothyroidotomy 27
    USG-guided 28
Cricothyrotomy 188, 194, 194f
Critical care
    fellow, basic ultrasound physics for 4
    ultrasound 1, 65
    unit 57, 141
Critical pericardial effusion 193
Custom made probe sheaths 115
Cutaneous nerve, posterior 186

D

Dark ring-like structures 179
Deep needle procedure 188, 190
Deep vein thrombosis 83, 85

Dehydration 109
Diagnostic peritoneal lavage 142
Diaphragm 41, 146
    anatomy, normal 43*f*
    basic anatomy of 44*f*
    movements 43*f*
Diastasis 74
Diastolic dysfunction 75, 76, 78*f*, 80*f*
    progressive 76
Diastolic flow
    blunted 135
    reversal 133*f*, 135
Diastolic function, normal 75
Disaster management 141
Distensibility index 60
Distracting injuries 140
Diverticulitis 104
Doppler assessment 70*f*
Doppler ultrasound 13
Dorsal venous arch 161
Dorsalis pedis artery 165
Duplex scanning 13
Dyskinesia 73

E

E and A reversal 76*f*
Echocardiographic views, basic 49, 50*f*, 57
Echocardiography 65
Echogenic calcium deposits 107
Echogenicity 106
Eclampsia 107
Effusions, types of 41
Ejection fraction 60-62
    different values of 74*t*
Electrocardiography 80
Elliptical disks, stack of 61
Emphysema lines 35
Emphysematous pyelonephritis 112
End diastolic velocity 110, 127, 134
Endocardium, inward motion of 72
Endotracheal intubation 25
Endotracheal tube placement 20, 141
Enhancement artifact 16, 18*f*
Epicardium 193
Epiglottis 20
Equipment 160, 176
Esophageal intubation 26
Esophagus 20
Excessive lung water, B lines suggestive of 56*f*
Eye
    to examine pupils 119
    ultrasound of 119*f*
Eyeballing 72
    principles, basic 57

F

Fascia iliaca compartment analgesia 185
Fascia lata 185
Fascial layers 156
Fascicle, pattern-like 186
Fast and efast views 145*f*
Fat 5
Femoral artery 163, 164*f*, 165, 165*f*, 185, 186
    superficial 186
Femoral nerve 164*f*, 185
    block 186
Femoral triangle 164*f*
Femoral vein 86, 163, 164, 164*f*, 165*f*, 173, 185
    position for scanning 86*f*
    right 87*f*
Fibrous tissue 106
Filling phase, rapid 74
First-pass success, high degree of 188
Flank view, right 146
Flow within vessels 115
Fluid
    administration 31, 47
    around gallbladder 96
    color sign 41
    identification of 190
    mimics, presence of 190
Foley's catheterization 150
Foot and ankle surgeries 184
Footprint 6
Foreign body 156, 158
Four vessel angiography 136
Fractional shortening 61, 61*f*
Fractures 118, 156
Fungal infections 113

G

Gallbladder 93
    calculi 95
    capacity of 93
    dimensions 95*f*
    distension 95
    lumen 96
    pathology 93
    ultrasound of 93
    wall thickening 95
Gallstones 93
Gastroduodenal artery 98
Glasgow come scale 117
Glomerulonephritis 107, 111
Glove drains 115
Gluteus maximus
    lies 186
    muscle 183

Gosling's pulsatility index 134
Gout 107
Great saphenous vein 164, 165f

H

Heart 92
    rate 64, 110
Hematoma 113, 167
Hemolytic-uremic syndrome 107
Hemopericardium, circulation assess for 142
Hemoperitoneum, circulation assess for 142
Hemothorax 142, 145, 155, 167
    circulation access for 142
Hepatic artery 98, 116
Hepatic veins, accessory 116
Hepatorenal space 146
Hepatorenal syndrome 111
High frequency probe 189
Hockey stick probe 176
Hunter's canal 163
Hydronephrosis 108, 113
    grades of 109f
    severe 109f
    with stent, severe 110f
Hyoid bone 158
Hypercontractile heart 60
Hyperechoic
    interface 176
    rim 176
    structure 186
    tissue, intervening 176
    vocal ligament 22f
Hyperkinesia 73
Hyperparathyroidism 107
Hypoechogenic renal cortex 107
Hypoechoic vocalis muscle 22f
Hypokinesia 72
    right ventricle free wall 91f
Hypoxemia 57

I

Infection 111
    presence of 190
Inferior vena cava 38, 52, 54f, 56, 83, 84f, 97-99, 152
    diameter variation 54
    long-axis view of 53f
    size 54
Information, basic 31
Infraclavicular approach brachial plexus block 180f
Infraclavicular fossa 179
Infragluteal approach 186

Infragluteal region 186
Inspired oxygen, fraction of 45
Intensive care unit 57, 93
Intercostal space 192
Internal jugular vein, anatomic variations of 165f
Interscalene block 177
Interstitial nephritis, acute 107
Intestinal obstruction 104
Intra-abdominal injury 142
Intracranial pressure 117, 121, 123f, 142
    estimations 132
Intraneural injections 175
Intraperitoneal hemorrhage 190
Intravascular filling, circulation access 142
Intravascular injections 175
Invasive intracranial monitors 117
Ipsilateral chest 192
Ischial tuberosity 183
Isovolumetric relaxation 74
IVC distensibility index 54

J

Jellyfish sign 41
Jugular vein
    cannulation, internal 176
    external 163
    internal 163, 173

K

Kidney
    disease
        acute 110
        chronic 107, 110
    echogenic nature of 106
    injury, acute 105-107, 108b, 111b
    left 149
    right 146
Kissing sign 60
Kissing ventricle sign 60

L

Landmark technique 173
Laryngeal mask airway placement 20
Lateral in-plane technique 173
Lateral resolution 10f
Left atrium 50, 51, 53, 68, 72
Left ventricle 62
    eyeballing of 62

Left ventricular
    ejection fraction 60
    end-diastolic area 60
        assessment of 60
    function
        assessment of 60, 73
            grading of 62t
        internal diameter
            end diastole 61
            end systole 61
        myocardium, 17-segment model of 73f
        outflow tract 51
Leg raising, passive 58
Lens 118
    dislocations 118
Lienorenal space 149
Life-threatening injuries 140
Linear transducer 161f
Liver 146
    disease 116
    pathologies of 116
    transplant patient 115
        ultrasound in 116
    ultrasound 115
Local anesthetic, make sure 190
Long bone fractures 158
Longitudinal scans 175
Loss of aeration, quantification of 46t
Lower limb
    blocks 183
    compression ultrasound 91
    deep veins of 164f
    venous ultrasound 86
Lumbar plexus 176
    branches of 183
Lumbar puncture 137, 188
    compared 194
    ultrasound-guided 194, 195f
Lumen, complete obliteration of 89f
Lung 92
    aeration 45
    anatomy of normal 34f
    comets 35
    consolidation 45
    in pneumothorax 38
    lower part of 146
    normal 32
    parenchyma, hepatization of 38
    point 39, 39f
        location of 39f
    pulse 38
    sliding, presence of 192
    sonography 31
        protocol 47
    ultrasound 31, 33f, 44, 47, 55, 91
    water component, extravascular 45

Lymph nodes 102
Lymphoceles 113

M

M mode 11
    PLAX view 12f
Magnetic resonance imaging 25
Maxillary sinus 124f
    haziness, complete left 125f
    left 124f
McConnell's sign 91
Mechanical ventilation, controlled 59
Medial cord 180
Medial scalene 178
Medulla 106
Medullary nephrocalcinosis 107
    causes of 107b
Medullary sponge kidney 107
Mesenteric artery, superior 83, 98
Mesenteric vein, superior 101
Metastasectomy 115
Mickey mouse sign 165f
Microconvex 7, 8f
Milk-alkali syndrome 107
Mitral annulus, longitudinal motion of 72
Mitral flow 80
Mitral regurgitation 69
    chronic 69
    severe 70f
Mitral stenosis 68, 69f, 70f
Mitral valve
    annulus, tissue Doppler imaging of 78
    inflow 74
        normal 75f
Monofascicular nerves, small 176
Morison's pouch 146
Muscle 5, 156
Muscularis propria 103
Musculocutaneous nerve 181
    block 182
Musculoskeletal injuries 156
Myeloma
    kidney 107
    multiple 107
Myocardium, thickening of 72

N

Nasal fracture 157
Neck and upper limb, major veins of 163f
Neck region plaque 126f
Necrosis 102
    areas of 100

Needle entry, angle of 189
Needle, localization of 190
Nephrogenic diabetes insipidus 109
Nerve 164
    block
        failures of 175
        perspective toward 187
        procedure for 178, 180
        ultrasound guided 175
    identification 175
    location, median 182*f*
    real-time objective 187
    ultrasound guided 177
Neurocritical care setting, ultrasound in 117
Neurotrauma 156, 158
Neurovascular bundle 156
Noncardiogenic pulmonary edema 46
Nonfunctioning obstructed kidney 109

O

Obesity 85, 160
Operation theaters 141
Optic nerve 118
    injury 156
    sheath 121, 122
        diameter 121, 122, 123*f*, 142
        dilated 123*f*
Orbital trauma, left 120*f*
Overdistended bladder 109

P

Pain, minimal 175
Pancreas
    head of 98
    locating 101*f*
    normal 98*f*
    tail of 98
    transverse view of 99*f*
    ultrasound of 93, 97
Pancreatic pseudocyst 101*f*
Pancreatic region 99
Pancreatitis 100*f*
    acute 99
    severe 107
Papillary necrosis 107
Paracentesis
    mechanical complications of 190
    needle 188, 190
    ultrasound-guided 190, 191*f*
Paradoxical motion 90
Paradoxical systolic motion 90

Parasternal short-axis view 52, 52*f*
Parenchyma 106, 107
Peak systolic
    velocity 110, 134
    volume 127
Pelvic 145
    longitudinal view 152*f*
    view 149
Pelvis and renal parenchyma 112*f*
Penetrating trauma 144
Percutaneous cricothyroidotomy 27
Percutaneous dilatational tracheostomy, ultrasound guidance during 26
Percutaneous kidney biopsy 113*f*
Percutaneous nephrostomy 113
Percutaneous renal biopsy 113
Percutaneous tracheostomy 188, 194*f*
    bronchoscopy guided 27
    safety of 194
    ultrasonography guided 27
    ultrasound guided 27, 194
Pericardial fluid
    accumulation, largest 193
    distribution of 193
    presence of 193
Pericardiocentesis 188, 193*f*
    ultrasound guided 193
Pericardium 193
Pericholecystic fluid 96
Perigraft fluid collection, drainage of 113
Peripancreatic collection, identification of 100
Peripartum hemorrhage 107
Peripheral venous access 173
Peristalsis 102
Piezoelectric crystal arrangement 6
Pleura, appearances of normal 32
Pleural effusion, sonographic appearance of 40*f*
Pleural sliding sign 33
Pleural space, left 149
Pneumonia, ventilator-associated 45
Pneumothorax 39*f*, 142, 155, 167
    diagnosis of 38
    procedure-related 192
Popliteal area 184
Popliteal artery 88*f*, 183, 186
Popliteal sciatic nerve 183*f*
Popliteal vein 87, 88*f*
    scanning 87*f*
Portal vein 84*f*, 101
    identification of 96
    undivided right 94
Positive end-expiratory pressure 25, 44
Posterolateral alveolar syndrome 47
Posterolateral pleural syndrome 47

Posterolaterally biceps femoris 186
Postextubation stridor 28
Pouch of Douglas 149, 151
Pre-Conception and Pre-Natal Diagnostic Techniques Act 2
Pregnancy, complications of 107
Pregnant uterus 190
Prerenal azotemia 111
Probe 5, 102
   and scan 145
   choice of 189
   placement 94
   positions 32, 32f
   sterility 190
   sterilization, different methods of 191f
Profunda femoris artery 186
Propagation velocities 5f
Proximal humerus 177
Proximal isovelocity surface area 68
Pseudoaneurysm 100
Pseudocyst 102
   late phase 100
Pulmonary artery 90, 91
   occlusion pressure, low 47
   systolic pressure 72
Pulmonary embolism 83, 85, 88, 90, 91
   evaluation of 57
Pulmonary venous flow 80
Pulsatile flow 167f
Pulsatility index 127
Pulse
   drops 110
   index continuous cardiac output 45
   wave 49
      Doppler 13, 66, 67f, 130, 166
Puncture 171
Pupil
   and reaction 119
   dilated 121f
Pyonephrosis 108
Pythagoras theorem 170f

Q

Quad sign 40

R

Radial artery 165
   cannulation 173
Randomized study comparing point-of-care 190
Reaeration, quantification of 46t
Real-time

fashion 188
methods 189
technique 168
Red Doppler signal 130
Reflection 8, 9f
Reflector scattering strength 14
Refraction 10
Regional anesthesia 175
   part of 175
Regional trauma 141
Regional wall motion abnormality 72
Relaxation, abnormal 79f
Renal anatomy, basic 106f
Renal tubular acidosis 107
Renal vein 98
Respiratory distress syndrome, acute 35
Restrictive pattern 80f
Retina 118
Retroperitoneal fibrosis 109
Retroperitoneal hemorrhage 85
Retrouterine pouch 149
Retrovesical pouch 149
Reverberation artifact 15f
Rib fractures 158f
Right atrium 50, 53, 56, 68, 72
Right upper quadrant 144-146, 147f
Right ventricular
   apex 195
   dilatation 90, 90f
   ejection fraction 65
   function, assessment of 64
   hypokinesia 90
   studies for dysfunction 57
   systolic pressure 72
Ring down artifact 16, 17f
Roentgenograms 140

S

Sacral plexus 183
   branches of 183
Safe puncture 41
Saphenous nerve block 183
Sarcoidosis 107
Scalene muscles 177
Scanning medium 162f
Schmidt group 116
Sciatic and femoral blocks 183
Sciatic nerve 183, 185
   block 183, 184, 186
Seashore sign 33, 34f, 39f
Segmental portal hypertension syndrome 100
Seldinger technique 170, 171
Semilunar tracheal ring, transverse view of 24f

Semimembranosus muscle 184
Sepsis 107
Septal position, abnormal 90
Septate effusion 41
Shock, rapid ultrasound in 92
Short axis technique 170f
Short axis view 164
Shred sign 37f, 38
Sickle cell disease 107
Simpson's method 73
Simpson's rule, modified 61
Sine wave 4
Sinus
    normal 123
    visualization of 122
Sinusogram 124
    complete 125f
Sinusoid sign 40
Skin 156
Soft tissue 5, 189
Sound wave 4
Spleen 149
Splenic vein 98
Split liver transplants harvests 116
Starry night appearance 41
Static technique 168
Stenotic lesions 130
Sterile gels 160
Sterile gloves 160
Sterile probe covers 160
Sterile transducer cover 189, 190
Sternocleidomastoid muscle 177, 178
Stomach, assessment of 28
Strap muscle 22f
Stratosphere sign 38, 39f
Stroke volume 49, 55, 62, 64
Subarachnoid hemorrhage 2
Subclavian
    artery 179, 180
    vein 163, 173
Subcostal view 53f
Submucosa 103
Superinfection 100
Superior vena cava 58
Supine position 180, 181
Supraclavicular fossa 178
Swelling, develops 119
Systemic vascular resistance 110
Systolic flows, sharp 135

T

Target sign 168, 170f
TCD tracings 130f, 131f

Tegaderm 122
Temporal resolution 10
Tendons 156
Thoracentesis, ultrasound guided 192
Thoracocentesis 188
Thrombectomy 112
Thrombosed veins 160
Thrombosis 100
Thrombus formation 116
Thyroid
    cartilage 20
        inverted V-shaped 22
        transverse section through 22f
    gland 23
Tissue 8
    Doppler 13, 64, 80
    Doppler mode 14
    harmonic imaging 13
Trachea, determine position of 141
Tracheal rings 20
Tracheal sign, double 26
Transabdominal ultrasound 116
Transcranial Doppler 117, 127, 130, 158
Transducer 6f
    in neck, orientation of 21
Transvenous pacing, ultrsound-guided 195f
Trauma surgeons 141
Traumatic procedures 194
Trendelenburg position 168
Tricuspid annular
    motion 64
    plane systolic excursion 64
Tricuspid annulus peak systolic velocity 64
    measurement of 65f
Tricuspid regurgitation 72, 72f
Tuberculosis 107
Tubular necrosis, acute 107, 111
Tumor 113

U

Ulnar artery 165
Ultrasonography 45, 140
    guidance 188
Ultrasound 4, 8, 28, 47, 94, 140, 160
    appearance 21, 98
    assistance 190
    beam 190
        shape 6
    findings 179, 180
    guidance increased 192
    guided cannulation, technique of 166
    guided technique 173
    image 189
        utilized technique 173

modes of 11
monitor 168
point of care 20, 57, 188, 190
role of 141
scan 177
use of 83
vision, advanced under direct 189
Upper airway, applied sonoanatomy of 20
Upper extremity blocks 177
Upper limb, veins of 162*f*
Upper quadrant, left 145, 148, 148*f*, 150*f*
Urinary bladder 153*f*
Urine leaks 113
Urinoma abscesses 113
Urinomas 113

V

Valves, Doppler evaluation of 65
Valvular lesion 67
Vascular access, ultrasound guided 160
Vascular injuries 116
Vascular structures, left back 116
Vasculotoxic snake bite 107
Vasospasm 118, 132
    diagnosis 132
    mild-moderate 132
    severe 132
Vein 164, 167*f*
    appear anechoic 166
    wall, tenting of 169*f*
Velocity, measurement of 55*f*
Velocity-time integral, measurement of 63*f*
Vena contracta 66, 68*f*
Ventilation, controlled 59
Ventricle, geometry of 72
Vesicoureteric reflux 109
Vessel, course of 168
Visceral pleura 40
Vitreous humor 118
Vocal cord 20
    visualization 21
Volume responsiveness using ultrasonography, assessment of 54
Volume status, assessment of 57

W

Water 5
Wave Doppler, continuous 13, 14, 66, 66*f*, 70, 72*f*
Wet lung profiles 36*f*
Wire-in-needle technique 173

www.ingramcontent.com/pod-product-compliance
Ingram Content Group UK Ltd.
Pitfield, Milton Keynes, MK11 3LW, UK
UKHW052020190225
455332UK00001B/11